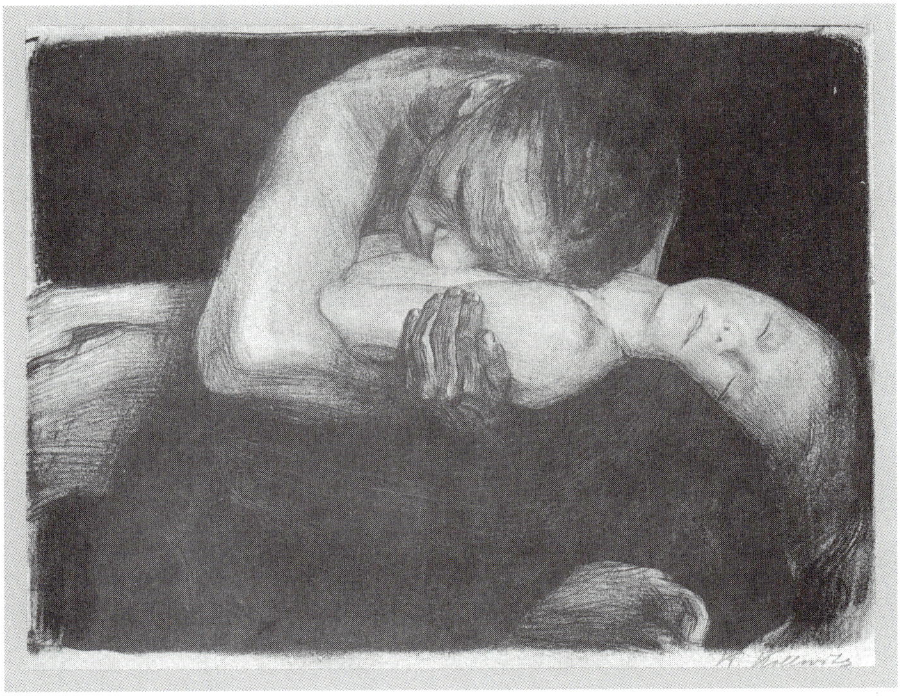

Front cover: Käthe Kollwitz, Pietá, Rosenwald Collection, © 1993 National Gallery of Art, Washington, DC.

THE CONTINUING CHALLENGE OF TUBERCULOSIS

Office of Technology Assessment
United States Congress

Recommended Citation:

U.S. Congress, Office of Technology Assessment, *The Continuing Challenge of Tuberculosis*, OTA-H-574 (Washington, DC: U.S. Government Printing Office, September 1993).

For sale by the U.S. Government Printing Office
Superintendent of Documents, Mail Stop: SSOP, Washington, DC 20402-9328
ISBN 0-16-041966-2

Foreword

After having declined for 30 years, the overall incidence of tuberculosis in the United States has been on the rise since the mid-1980s. In some communities, the problem is extremely serious, compounding other social ills, including AIDS, homelessness, drug abuse, and poverty. Particularly disturbing is the emergence of multidrug-resistant tuberculosis (MDR-TB). MDR-TB has been directly linked to inappropriate and incomplete treatment, which in turn has been linked, in part, to a lack of resources to ensure the proper delivery of tuberculosis services.

At at a time when the Nation is focused on health care reform, the threat of TB reminds us of the importance of maintaining a strong public health infrastructure. The Federal Government has a long history of providing resources and leadership to State and local health authorities in the control of TB. However, only in the past few years has the government begun to restore funding to TB programs that were cut during the 1970s and early 1980s.

OTA's report synthesizes current understanding of TB in the United States, including the extent of the disease, the state of research of new preventive, diagnostic, and therapeutic technologies to aid in its control, and the delivery of effective TB services. The report also provides an overview of Federal involvement in these activities.

It was initiated in response to requests from three committees of Congress: the House Committee on Energy and Commerce's Subcommittee on Health and the Environment, the House Committee on Government Operations' Subcommittee on Human Resources and Intergovernmental Relations, and the Senate Committee on Labor and Human Resources.

OTA was assisted in the study by a group of public health leaders from academia, industry, government, and public interest groups who met in a workshop convened by OTA in March 1993. A large number of other experts provided detailed reviews of multiple drafts.

OTA gratefully acknowledges the contribution of these individuals. As with all OTA reports, the final responsibility for the content of these assessments rests with OTA.

Roger C. Herdman, Director

Workshop Participants

Alan Bloch
Medical Officer
Surveillance and Epidemiology Branch
Centers for Disease Control and Prevention
U.S. Department of Health and Human Services
Atlanta, GA

Barry Bloom
Professor
Department of Microbiology and Immunology
Albert Einstein College of Medicine
Yeshiva University
Bronx, NY

Wafaa El-Sadr
Director
Division of Infectious Diseases
Harlem Hospital Center
New York, NY

Larry Gostin
Executive Director
American Society of Law, Medicine and Ethics
Boston, MA

Margaret Hamburg
Commissioner of Health
New York City Department of Health
New York, NY

Jeffrey Levi
Director
Government Affairs
AIDS Action Council
Washington, DC

Joan Otten
Director
Office of Tuberculosis Control
Jackson Memorial Hospital
Miami, FL

Lee Reichman
President
American Lung Association
New York, NY

Gisela Schecter
Tuberculosis Controller
Tuberculosis Control Division
Department of Public Health
City and County of San Francisco
San Francisco, CA

Peter Selwyn
Associate Director
AIDS Program
Yale-New Haven Hospital
New Haven, CT

Virginia Shubert
Director of Advocacy and Public Policy
Housing Works, Inc.
New York, NY

Jane Sisk
Professor
School of Public Health
Columbia University
New York, NY

Jeffrey Starke
Assistant Professor
Department of Pediatrics
Baylor College of Medicine
Houston, TX

OTA appreciates and is grateful for the valuable assistance and thoughtful critiques provided by the participants in OTA's workshop on Policy Issues in the Control of Tuberculosis, March 23, 1993. The workshop participants do not, however, necessarily approve, disapprove, or endorse this report. OTA assumes full responsibility for the report and the accuracy of its contents.

Project Staff

Clyde J. Behney
Assistant Director, OTA
Health, Life Sciences, and the Environment

ADMINISTRATIVE STAFF

Beckie Erickson
Office Administrator

Daniel B. Carson
PC Specialist

Carolyn Martin
Word Processing Specialist

Eric L. Gille
Secretary

PUBLISHING STAFF

Mary Lou Higgs
Manager, Publishing Services

Denise Felix
Production Editor

Dorinda Edmondson
Typographer

Christine Onrubia
Graphic Designer

PROJECT STAFF

MICHAEL E. GLUCK
Project Director

JULIA T. OSTROWSKY
Principal Contractor

Sharon Y. Hamilton
Research Analyst[1]

Arna M. Lane
Research Analyst

Contractors

Sue Etkind
Massachusetts Department of Public Health
Boston, MA

Lynn Powers
Editorial Consultant
Alexandria, VA

[1] From August 1992 to May 1993

Contents

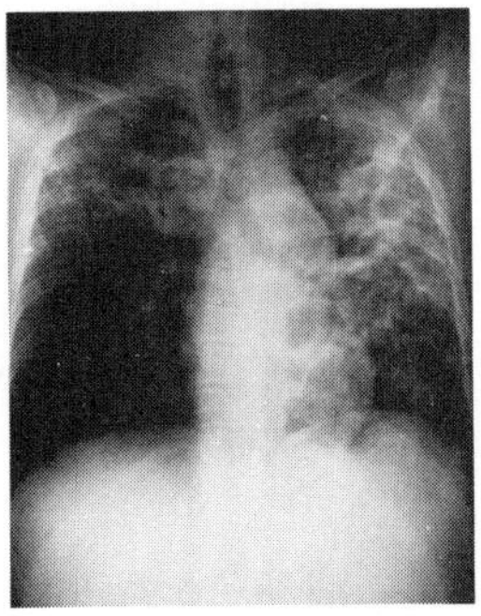

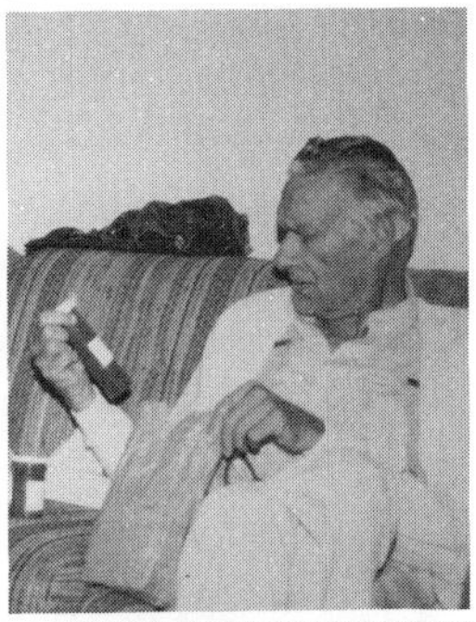

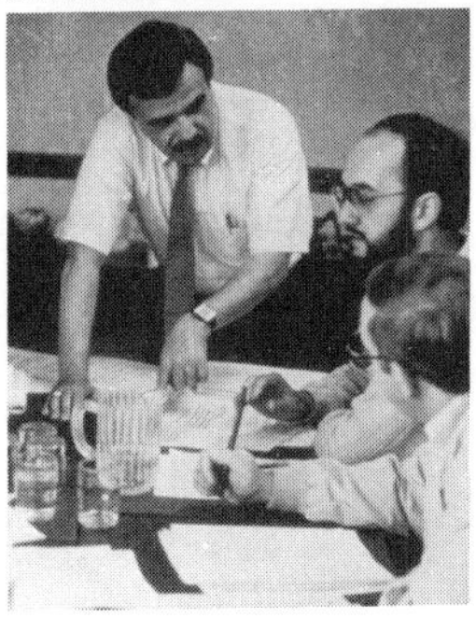

Summary and Policy Options 1

Tuberculosis (TB) is a contagious disease that has killed millions of people worldwide over the centuries. The lack of a reliable cure prior to this century and TB's perceived randomness made it a common theme in literature and a metaphor for larger social and political ills (84,299). Today, TB continues to be a public health threat in the United States. After decreasing in the country as a whole for many decades, rates of TB disease are again on the rise. In some communities, particularly among economically disadvantaged groups, TB rates have consistently remained high.

Recent trends in the incidence of TB have been linked, in part, to decreases in public health investment over the last two decades (45,46,176). Other factors associated with the resurgence of TB include the human immunodeficiency virus (HIV) epidemic, foreign birth, substance abuse, poverty, and homelessness. An important complication is the emergence of TB strains resistant to the most commonly used anti-TB drugs.

Unchecked, these recent trends in TB represent a serious threat to communities already saddled with poor health, poverty, and other social problems. Furthermore, this disease could become a additional major burden to the Nation's health care system.

Unlike the TB of past centuries, however, today's TB is amenable to human intervention. We know how it is spread. We know how to cure it, and we know how to prevent it. Although the primary governmental responsibility for controlling TB in the

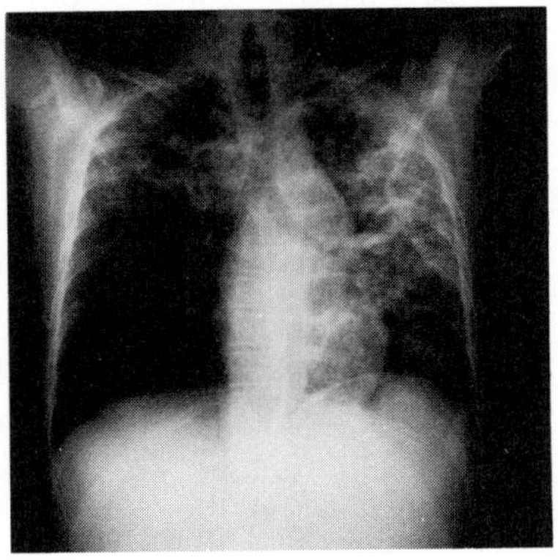

NOTE: Because of the large amount of material synthesized to produce this report, most citations to the literature underlying this summary chapter are omitted. However, the detailed analysis presented in subsequent chapters is fully referenced, and the summary in this chapter closely follows the organization of the subsequent chapters. References to ideas that are found only in this chapter are given where they occur.

United States falls to State and local authorities, the Federal Government has had, and continues to have, a substantial role in eliminating this disease. This report synthesizes scientific understanding of TB in the United States in 1993 and considers the Federal role in its control.

SCOPE OF THE OTA REPORT

Three congressional committees requested this report: the Subcommittee on Health and the Environment of the House Committee on Energy and Commerce, the Subcommittee on Human Resources and Intergovernmental Relations of the House Committee on Government Relations, and the Senate Committee on Labor and Human Resources. The report provides information on the problems posed by TB that Congress can use in considering alternative Federal policy responses. Although the report gives an overview of the direction and magnitude of Federal involvement in TB control and considers options for Congress, the report does not evaluate in detail the effectiveness of specific programs in individual communities or Federal agencies. Another congressional research agency, the General Accounting Office (GAO), is currently evaluating the effectiveness of efforts to control TB in several communities hit hard by the disease (183).

One-third of the world's population is infected with the organism that causes TB. With significant migration to the United States by people from countries with high levels of TB, foreign birth is a risk factor for the disease in this country. Hence, controlling TB abroad could have some impact on levels of TB in the United States. Although this report briefly considers the Federal Government's support of international organizations involved in TB control in developing countries, it focuses on TB as it occurs in the United States.

Tuberculosis, Health Care Reform, and Public Health Investments

As policymakers focus on health care reform, the analysis in this report indicates that TB will not disappear with improved access and better cost control of health care services alone. Even with universal access to medical services, a change in the organization and financing of health care will not, in and of itself, eliminate the need for Federal funding and coordination of the infrastructure to conduct education, surveillance, screening, diagnosis, research, and even treatment.

Furthermore, TB control is an exercise in vigilance. With an estimated one-third of the world's population infected with TB and the relative mobility of people in and out of the United States through immigration and tourism, the complete eradication of tuberculosis from this country is unlikely in the foreseeable future. In addition, people infected with the organism that causes TB now may progress to active disease many years in the future, after the current epidemic is brought under control. Nevertheless, TB control measures can lower disease rates and minimize the public health threat posed by the disease. Achieving such a goal will require a properly targeted and sustained effort. Once this goal is achieved, continued investment to identify, treat, and prevent TB will be necessary to maintain low disease rates. The current resurgence in TB is evidence that this last lesson was not learned in the past. Even in the last year, the Centers for Disease Control and Prevention (CDC) noted its own failure to implement recent TB control recommendations, due largely to a lack of resources (337).

What Is TB?

In 1882, the German scientist Robert Koch identified a species of bacteria, *Mycobacterium tuberculosis* (*M.tb.* or tubercle bacilli) as the cause of TB. There are two general stages of the disease: tuberculous infection (or "latent TB") and active tuberculosis. Individuals with tuberculous infection are asymptomatic and not contagious, whereas individuals with active TB can be symptomatic and contagious. Tuberculous infection is necessary to develop TB, but overall only 10 percent of those with the infection ever develop active TB. Risk is higher for children and for people with HIV and other disorders that impair immunity. In immunocompetent individuals, the immune system is usually able to contain most tuberculous infections. A tuberculin skin test, which uses a substance known as purified protein derivative (PPD), is used to detect tuberculous infection. In most immunocompetent people with the infection, this test produces a small raised area on the skin within 48 to 72 hours of administration.

While active TB can attack various parts of the body, pulmonary TB is the most common and leads to the destruction of lung tissue and frequently death if untreated. Symptoms include weakness, fever, chest pain, cough, and when a small blood vessel is eroded, bloody sputum. Active TB can also occur in other parts of the body, with the brain (TB meningitis) being the most serious. TB outside the lungs is more likely to occur among children and people with HIV.

What Is the Risk of TB Infection?

People with TB are contagious when they expel airborne particles containing viable tubercle bacilli through, for example, coughing, singing, speaking, or sneezing. The likelihood of infection depends mainly on the:

- Probability of coming into contact with someone with contagious, active TB;
- Closeness or intimacy of the contact;
- Duration of the contact;
- Number of viable bacilli present in the air;
- Susceptibility of the uninfected case; and
- Environmental conditions (e.g., volume of airspace, ventilation with outside air, relative humidity, presence of sunlight).

Health care workers (HCWs) are at increased risk of infection, particularly if they perform cough-inducing medical procedures on patients with active pulmonary TB and if they work in environments with inadequate infection control measures.

Casual contact with an infectious person—i.e. with active, untreated TB—in a public place such as a movie theater or subway is unlikely to lead to infection, although the risk is not zero. Although infection occurs at a specific point in time when an infectious particle is inhaled, the longer the exposure, the greater the likelihood an infectious particle will be inhaled. Hence, exposure to an infectious person over a period of months is usually necessary for transmission to occur.

In general, less than 30 percent of household members become infected while living with an infectious person, but the risk is highly variable. Under extraordinary circumstances (when the concentration of airborne infectious particles is unusually high), exposures as brief as 2 hours have reportedly led to infection.

Adequate anti-microbial or anti-tuberculosis treatment can reduce the infectiousness of drug-susceptible TB within days. Although the exact amount of time needed to eliminate the infection completely varies by patient, it is about 6 months or longer. While there is no evidence that drug-resistant TB is more contagious than drug-susceptible TB, delays in diagnosis and treatment allow patients to remain infectious for a longer period of time, thus increasing chances of infecting others.

Trends in the Incidence of Active TB

Between 1953, when the Public Health Service (PHS) first implemented a national reporting system for active TB cases, and 1984, the number of annually reported cases declined 74 percent from 84,304 (53 per 100,000 population) to

Figure 1-1—Reported Tuberculosis Cases in the United States, 1953-92

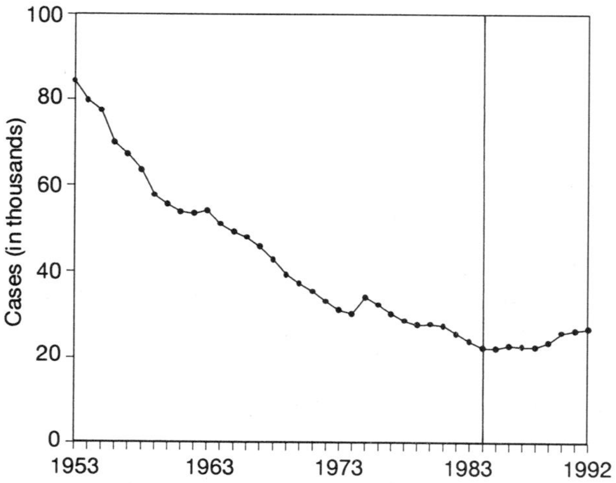

SOURCE: Office of Technology Assessment, 1993, based on data from U.S. Department of Health and Human Services, Public Health Service, Centers for Disease Control and Prevention, 1992.

22,255 (9.4 per 100,000). Beginning in 1985, this decline slowed and then reversed (figure 1-1). The number of new cases reported in 1992 was 26,673 (10.5 per 100,000), a 20 percent increase over 1985.

The Changing Demographics of TB

Over the years, TB has gradually shifted from a disease broadly distributed over the whole population to one that is more narrowly concentrated among certain portions of the population. Although the rapid increase in the overall number of new cases suggests a potential threat to the population as a whole, the current concentrations of the disease offer TB-control experts and policymakers a guide in targeting resources for controlling TB. Groups with particularly high rates of TB can be described according to geography, race, ethnicity, and factors causally related to the disease.

Heavy Concentrations in Certain Parts of the Country

The most populous States have the largest number of cases. In 1991, over half of all TB cases came from California, New York, Texas, Florida, and Illinois. Urban areas with populations over 250,000 contained 18 percent of the country's population but 43 percent of its new TB cases in that year. The number of new TB cases per 100,000 of population in the South has always been above the national average, although New York, Hawaii, and California have the highest rates. Among cities, Atlanta (76.4 per 100,000), Newark (71.8 per 100,000), New York (50.3 per 100,000), Miami (48.5 per 100,000), and San Francisco (46.0 per 100,000) had the highest case rates[1] during 1991.

Accounting for 14 percent of the total number of new TB cases reported in the United States during 1991 and with a TB case rate five times the national average, New York City alone has a significant, concentrated portion of the Nation's entire TB problem. In one part of the city, Central Harlem, the case rate was 169.2 per 100,000 in 1989 and has never dipped below 52 during the 40 years that data have been kept (45).

Heavy Concentrations Among Minorities and the Young

Within a given geographic area, certain demographic groups are more likely than others to produce new cases of TB. In 1991, 71 percent of new cases occurred in racial and ethnic minorities. Hispanic Americans, Black Americans, and Americans of Asian or Pacific Island[2] origin showed relatively large increases in TB during the 1985-91 period. Although the risk of TB in adults increased with age, this pattern was not consistent across different racial and ethnic groups. Among white, non-Hispanic Americans, most TB cases occurred among elderly people, while among

[1] A "case rate" is defined as the number of cases of active TB diagnosed in a given year per 100,000 population.

[2] Terms used to describe these demographic groups are those used in the original studies from which the epidemiologic findings are drawn.

Black and Hispanic Americans, the bulk occurred in the 25 to 44 year-old age group.

Rates of increase have been disproportionately high among children; this trend is also concentrated among racial and ethnic minorities, who accounted for 86 percent of all childhood cases in 1991. Childhood cases of TB are strong evidence of recent transmission of the disease, suggesting contact with other infectious individuals in the community and possibly more, undetected cases of infection. High rates of TB among immigrants and increases in TB among parents in the 25 to 44 age group may account for the observed increases among children. Furthermore, children infected now could suffer active disease years in the future.

High Rates Among Immigrants, Prisoners, Drug Users, Migrant Workers, and Homeless People

Being born outside the United States, being homeless, a substance abuser, being incarcerated, or being a migrant worker is a risk factor for tuberculous infection. In addition, being coinfected with HIV increases one's risk of progressing from infection to active disease. The overlap among these groups reinforces the concentration of TB within the United States population and the particular risk for members of these groups.

Given the high prevalence of TB infection in many other parts of the world (171), a large percentage of new TB cases in the United States occur among individuals born elsewhere (27 percent in 1991). Among homeless populations, several studies have found latent TB infection to be as high as 50 percent. Impaired immunity due to poor overall health, substance abuse, or HIV infection may cause homeless people with tuberculous infection to progress to active disease. In addition, homeless shelters can generate new transmissions, due to crowding and poor ventilation. Twenty percent of newly diagnosed TB cases in New York City in 1991 were homeless.

Substance-abusing populations overlap with other groups at high risk of TB, especially with homeless and HIV-infected people.

The prevalence of TB in prisons is related to the close living quarters, poor ventilation, and other risk factors that inmates may possess. In some States, epidemiologists have estimated that TB may be as much as 6 to 11 times more prevalent among prisoners than among the general population. Prison populations comprise other groups at high risk of TB—drug users, HIV-infected people, and individuals homeless prior to incarceration. Persons with active TB in prisons cannot only spread the disease among other prisoners, but they also place at-risk prison staff and family or friends with whom they have close contact upon their release.

Among migrant workers, lack of access to health services and lack of adequate working and housing conditions are believed to contribute to the heightened risk of TB as noted among some limited recent studies. Many members of this group are also poor, minorities, foreign born, or former homeless shelter residents.

People With HIV Have High TB Rates

HIV is the pathogen that causes acquired immunodeficiency syndrome (AIDS). Because HIV-related immunosuppression impairs the body's ability to fight a tuberculous infection, individuals infected with both tubercle bacilli and HIV are estimated to have a risk of as high as 8 percent per year of progressing rapidly to active TB disease, compared with a 10 percent lifetime risk for HIV-negative individuals.

Epidemiologic evidence has consistently shown a higher prevalence of TB among individuals with AIDS compared with the general population, even after adjustment for age, race, and sex. In addition, more than one-half of deaths with TB in individuals 20 to 49 years old appear to occur in people who also have AIDS.[3]

Multidrug-Resistant Tuberculosis

When a patient takes TB medication erratically or when an inadequate combination of drugs is prescribed, active, infectious TB can recur in a form resistant to one or more of the drugs used in the original treatment.[4] As described later in this chapter and in detail in chapter 4, cases of MDR-TB are far more difficult and costly to treat than drug-sensitive TB, and can be fatal despite the best available treatment. CDC began regularly collecting drug susceptibility data on each reported case of TB in 1993, a practice done periodically with surveys prior to 1986.

Preliminary data from a 1991 CDC survey indicate that drug resistant TB cases have been reported in all regions of the country, but are most heavily concentrated in a few States. Cases resistant to at least one drug were found in 36 States and to two or more drugs in 13 States. Of the cases found to be resistant to the two most commonly used drugs, isoniazid (INH) and rifampin (RIF), over half were in New York City. In a separate study, 33 percent of the 466 TB cases reported in New York City during April 1991 were resistant to one or more drugs, and 19 percent were resistant to both INH and RIF.

Since 1990, there have been at least 9 outbreaks of MDR-TB among 297 individuals in prisons and hospitals. Most of these people were HIV-infected. As many as 89 percent of those with MDR-TB (including 6 health care workers and 1 prison guard) have died from their TB.[5] Delayed or inadequate infection control measures, premature discontinuation of patient isolation, delayed reporting of drug resistance, and lack of isolation facilities were major factors in the spread of MDR-TB in these institutions.

Three Strategies for TB Prevention

Under public policy discussion are three strategies for preventing the spread of TB—infection control, finding and offering preventive treatment to infected high-risk populations, and bacillus Calmette-Guérin (BCG) vaccination.

Infection Control

Although tuberculous infection has long been known as an occupational hazard for health care workers, and although there is some evidence that HCWs in some jobs (e.g. pulmonary medicine) are at greater risk than other HCWs, the actual magnitude of the risks have not been well documented in recent years.

CDC updated its guidelines for preventing TB transmission within hospitals in 1990 and is expected to do so again in the near future (79). The guidelines call for a "hierarchy of controls," including limiting exposure to the source of infection (through identification, respiratory isolation, and prompt treatment of infectious patients), implementing environmental measures, and using individual protective devices. None of these measures are believed to have been widely adopted by hospitals or other institutions.

Although implementing combinations of these measures appears to have been effective in ending the recent outbreaks, there are few data on the effectiveness of individual measures under conditions of actual use (79).[6] In practice, decisions

[3] Despite the prevalence of TB among those with HIV, *M.tb.* may represent only 10 percent of mycobacterial infections in this patient group. Non-tuberculous mycobacteria (e.g., *M. avium*) is very common among AIDS patients; these infections occur in later stages of AIDS (when CD4 cell counts are below $100/mm^3$), are untreatable, and may be fatal.

[4] Strains of TB treatable with available anti-TB medications are called "drug sensitive." Strains resistant to at least one anti-TB medication are called "drug-resistant." According to the CDC, strains resistant to, at least, isoniazid and rifampin are referred to as MDR-TB.

[5] It is unknown whether the high rate of mortality observed in these outbreaks applies to other HIV-infected populations or to HIV-negative individuals.

[6] CDC currently has some such research underway with plans to begin more in the future (see chapter 7).

about the adoption of individual measures depend not just on their efficacy in controlled experiments, but also on their feasibility given the physical characteristics of the relevant facility, the patient population, and available resources.

Another basic component of CDC's guidelines is achieving adequate ventilation, which can be difficult in modern facilities designed for energy conservation or in older buildings without central air circulation. New devices are under development to filter and recirculate air within individual rooms. Also, germicidal ultraviolet-C (UV-C) light has been advocated as an adjunct to ventilation controls, as have masks designed to fit tightly around the mouth and nose (called disposable particulate respirators); but ***data on the effectiveness of each under actual conditions of use are lacking.***

In 1992, the National Institute of Occupational Safety and Health (NIOSH), a part of the CDC, recommended that HCWs who come in contact with infectious TB patients should wear "powered air purifying respirators" (PAPRs), devices commonly employed in industrial settings to protect workers from toxic fumes and other substances. Other TB experts at CDC criticized the NIOSH recommendation, arguing that PAPRs are unnecessary and interfere with the provision of clinical care. TB experts outside of CDC report that these contradictory recommendations have caused confusion among HCWs, patients, and those charged with controlling infection in facilities with TB patients (304). The divergent recommendations may reflect the different missions of NIOSH and the rest of CDC. While NIOSH is mandated to seek zero occupational risk, the position of the others at CDC on PAPRs reflects an attempt to balance worker safety with the provision of feasible effective treatment to patients (79). Whatever the intent or impact of these recommendations, however, there is currently no evidence on the effectiveness of PAPRs.

Skin Testing and Preventive Treatment

For several decades, it has been theoretically possible to prevent most new cases of TB with available diagnostic and preventive treatment methods. As TB has retreated from the general population and become more concentrated among subset populations, such targeted efforts should have become more feasible. Indeed, CDC has long recommended screening for tuberculous infection among groups with high rates of TB, with HIV, or with other risk factors for developing active disease and INH preventive treatment (IPT) for those found to be infected. ***The ability to implement these recommendations has been limited largely by the availability of funding, other resources, and knowledge about the most cost-effective methods of providing these services to high-risk groups.***

In order to prescribe IPT, one must first detect a TB infection, usually with the PPD tuberculin skin test. For otherwise healthy people, the test detects an existing infection about 95 percent of the time with a variable false positive rate. For people with HIV and other immune deficiencies, the test is much less likely to detect tuberculous infection (due to a condition called anergy), reducing its effectiveness as a screening tool in these populations and thus limiting the use of IPT.

For those with tuberculous infection the preventive use of the anti-TB drug isoniazid (INH) has been shown in large, randomized clinical trials to be as much as 90 percent effective in eliminating the bacilli from the body and preventing subsequent development of active disease. Between 2 and 3 percent of adults over age 50 receiving INH develop liver inflammation that can lead to hepatitis if the drug is not stopped when blood tests reveal the condition.

BCG Vaccination

Since the early 1950s, the World Health Organization (WHO) has advocated widespread vaccination with BCG as a preventive measure against TB in countries with a high prevalence of the disease. Currently, about 70 percent of the world's children receive BCG. However, BCG has never been widely used in the United States due, in part, to controversy over its efficacy and low expected utility in populations in which the rate of TB transmission is relatively low.

BCG refers to several strains of bovine tubercle bacilli derived from a single strain produced about 70 years ago in France. One form of BCG is currently manufactured and sold with Food and Drug Administration (FDA) approval in the United States. Instead of preventing initial TB infection, BCG is believed to enhance the body's immune response to the infection and prevent the multiplication and dissemination of bacilli to various parts of the body.

Several studies, including randomized clinical trials, have produced estimates of the preventive efficacy of BCG that range from zero (or negative) to 80 percent. It is also unclear how long BCG might enhance immunity and whether HIV-related immunodeficiency inhibits the vaccines' usefulness. Attempts to interpret the existing data and understand the differing results continue. Some research does suggest that BCG may be more effective in preventing the more serious extrapulmonary forms of TB among children than in preventing the pulmonary forms of the disease. Although side effects are rare and data are insufficient to make actual risk estimates, there have been published case reports of BCG complications among HIV-infected individuals.

BCG vaccination may itself cause subsequent tuberculin skin tests to show up as positive for 3 to 5 years, thereby complicating public health efforts to detect actual infections and offer preventive treatment. ***Framed as a policy choice among alternative strategies for prevention, Federal policy in the United States has long favored strong infection control, skin testing, and preventive treatment. However, CDC does recommend selected use of the vaccine in high-risk infants and children for whom preventive treatment is infeasible or culturally unacceptable.***

Diagnosis of Active TB

At present, diagnosis of active TB is based on a combination of clinical symptoms, laboratory tests, and chest x-ray findings. Although these technologies have been generally adequate, their deficiencies have grown in the face of rising drug resistance and the need to prevent the rapid spread of TB among patients who have HIV or who live in congregate settings.

The TB skin test used for detecting tuberculous infection is considered inadequate for diagnosing active disease, partly because of its unreliability with immunocompromised and other sick people and with the minimum of 48 hours required for results. The initial diagnostic laboratory test is the sputum smear in which a sample of the patient's sputum is stained with a dye for acid fast bacilli (AFB) and is examined under a light microscope. However, only 50 to 80 percent of patients with active TB have positive sputum smears, and the rate may be even lower for people with HIV. Hence, negative smears cannot be used to rule out TB. Chest x-rays are also used to detect signs of the presence of TB in the lungs or the damage caused by the disease.

Definitive diagnosis of TB has been traditionally based on culturing and identifying tubercle bacilli from a patient's sputum, body fluids, or tissue in the laboratory. This test takes 3 to 6 weeks given the bacilli's slow rate of growth. A relatively new, automated, radiometric device (known by the trade name of BACTEC™) reduces testing time to about 10 days by measuring carbon dioxide given off by the tubercle bacilli. Other diagnostic technologies are under development.

Effective treatment depends on determining the susceptibility of a patient's TB to anti-tuberculosis drugs. Delayed diagnosis and drug susceptibility testing were considered to be one of the main factors contributing to the recent outbreaks of MDR-TB and continue to represent a major impediment in the control of TB. Conventional methods of drug susceptibility testing typically require 8 to 12 weeks. Newer radiometric techniques used with direct testing can determine susceptibility to the five first-line drugs within 3 weeks, although these tests are relatively expensive and not yet widely available.

Newer diagnostic technologies under study include a genetic technique called polymerase chain reaction (PCR) to amplify the amount of deoxyribonucelic acid (DNA) material specific to tubercle bacilli. PCR-based diagnosis has reportedly produced results in research conditions within 48 hours. However, PCR techniques currently carry a high risk of operator error, and TB diagnosis using this technology is not yet available for nonexperimental use (29,30).[7] A recently reported method uses the light-producing enzyme from fireflies to distinguish drug-resistant and drug-sensitive tubercule bacilli in 2 to 3 days. However, this technology has not yet been adapted for clinical use. Other quick diagnostic technologies are in various stages of development.

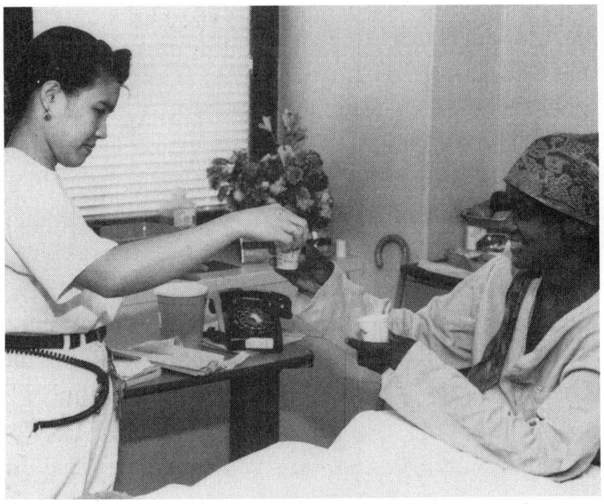

AMERICAN LUNG ASSOCIATION

Treatment of drug-susceptible TB involves taking three or four drugs together on a daily, two-, or three-time a week basis for 6 months. However, hospitalization is usually not necessary after a few weeks of treatment renders the patient noninfectious. Treatment of drug-resistant TB can involve more drugs for a longer period of time and potentially longer hospital stays.

Treatment of Active TB

The introduction of antibiotic drug treatment in the 1940s dramatically changed the practice and outcome of TB treatment. Over the past 20 years, no new drugs have replaced or supplemented the five main first-line drugs—INH, RIF, pyrazinamide (PZA), ethambutol (EMB), and streptomycin (SM)—although other drugs of lesser effectiveness and greater toxicity are available as second-line drugs. In addition, clinical research has permitted a better understanding of how drugs eliminate TB from the body as well as the refinement of drug treatment regimens.

Combinations of antimicrobial drugs with overlapping functions are used in current treatment regimens to attack tubercle bacilli in the body. Anti-tuberculous drugs are generally classified as bactericidal (producing rapid killing of bacilli) or sterilizing (killing the last surviving, slowly metabolizing bacilli over the long-term). INH is the major bactericidal drug. RIF and PZA are the most potent sterilizing drugs.

Current regimens usually consist of two phases and can, if taken fully, produce cure rates of 98 percent with relapses among less than 3 percent. During an initial 2-month bactericidal phase, the daily use of INH, RIF, PZA, and SM or EMB is intended to eliminate quickly the bulk of tubercle bacilli. During the second 4 to 5 month sterilizing phase, patients take INH and RIF on a daily schedule or a two- to three-time a week schedule to eliminate remaining bacilli. These drugs can cause side effects, the most serious of which is hepatitis, an inflammation of the liver.

By comparison, treatment of MDR-TB is longer, potentially more toxic, less effective, and significantly more costly. Drug regimens for MDR-TB are determined on a case-by-case basis using information on the patient's prior drug therapy, drug-susceptibility testing of the pa-

[7] One manufacturer, Hoffman LaRoche, offers this test as a service for laboratories that provide it with patient tissue samples; however, the cost is approximately $175 per specimen, making it relatively expensive (29,30).

tient's bacilli, and the patient's tolerance of adverse effects. Cases resistant to two or more of the first-line drugs would be treated with combinations of drugs selected from among the first- and second-line drugs, often for 18 to 24 months or longer.

The arsenal of second-line TB drugs includes: capreomycin, kanamycin, ethionamide, cycloserine, and p-aminosalicyclic acid. Reliable data to judge the effectiveness of these second-line drugs are lacking, but anecdotal experience suggests that they are much less effective and more likely to lead to serious toxic effects. Adjunctive surgery to remove heavily infected tissue (usually in the lung) is sometimes used as a last resort when drug treatment is inadequate in patients with localized pulmonary TB.

Current evidence suggests that drug-sensitive TB is curable in many individuals with HIV, even some with advanced stages of immunodeficiency. Most documented cases of treatment failure in patients with HIV have been linked with incomplete treatment or poor absorption of antituberculosis drugs. The major problems in treating TB in HIV-infected people are drug side effects and interactions with other treatments or conditions.

Recently, the FDA has worked with drug manufacturers to rectify shortages of some drugs. Public health officials have also expressed concern over increases in the price of antituberculosis drug treatments. Table 1-1 shows the results of a recent CDC survey of the prices paid by State and local health departments for drugs they purchase for two common TB drug regimens. Table 1-1 suggests drug price increases of about 9 percent per year on average between 1986 and 1992 for treating an uncomplicated case and about 12 percent per year for treating a patient resistant to INH and RIF.

Current research is focused on developing new drugs, shorter regimens, and better methods of drug delivery. A number of individual drugs are being investigated for anti-TB activity, but so far there is limited or no data about their efficacy and safety from controlled clinical trials. Among such drugs not yet approved for TB treatment in the United States are clofazamine and the classes of drugs known as quinolones, rifamycin derivatives, and phenazines.

Combination tablets containing INH and RIF (known by the trade name Rifamate™) are approved by the FDA but not widely used in the United States. In 1993, the FDA received an application to market Rifater™, a combination of INH, RIF, and PZA, in the United States. Implantable devices containing anti-TB drugs for slow release similar to the contraceptive Norplant™ are not yet ready for clinical evaluation. Immunotherapeutic approaches to treating TB are also under investigation.

Delivering TB Treatment

Because current TB treatment involves taking multiple drugs over many months, complete, appropriate treatment can be hard to achieve. Hence, the delivery of treatment is as important for TB control as is the arsenal of available drugs themselves. Current programs to deliver treatment and other TB services are heterogeneous and can vary across and with communities.

Data based on samples of TB case reports suggest that about 75 percent of U.S. patients being treated for TB complete treatment within a year and that 80 percent take their medication on a continuous basis. However, these national averages obscure wide variation among different areas of the country. For example, in the late 1980s, cities such as Chicago, New York, and the District of Columbia reported completion rates ranging from 54 to 60 percent, while Dallas, San Francisco, and El Paso had rates above 94 percent.

While much public discussion has focused on patient behavior as the cause of treatment failure, evidence suggests that the availability and quality of TB control services as well as prescription of optimal treatment regimens may be equally important in determining whether patients are cured.

Table 1-1—Trends in Drug Costs for Treating Tuberculosis in a 165 lb (75 kg) Patient, 1986-92: An Uncomplicated Case Versus a Case Resistant to INH and RIF[a]

***Uncomplicated case*:**

Drug	Daily dose	Duration	1986 cost	1990 cost	1992 cost
Isonizaid	300 mg	180 days	$ 5.04	$ 6.50	$ 8.50
Rifampin	600 mg	180 days	106.20	159.30	165.30
Pyrazinamide	25 mg/kg	60 days	98.00	160.00	179.20
			$209.24	**$325.80**	**$353.00**

Average annual percentage increase in cost, 1986-92: **9.1%**

***A case resistant to INH and RIF*:**

Drug	Daily dose	Duration	1986 cost	1990 cost	1992 cost
Pyrazinamide	25 mg/kg	540 days	$ 882.00	$1,440.00	$1,613.00
Ethambutol	15 mg/kg	540 days	690.00	1,246.00	1,610.00
Streptomycin	15 mg/kg	120 days	138.00	192.00	206.00
Ethionamide	20 mg/kg	540 days	890.00	1,458.00	1,691.00
Ciprofloxacin	1500 mg	540 days	NA	3,000.00	3,600.00
			$2,600.00	**$7,338.00**	**$8720.00***

Average annual percentage increase in cost, 1986-92 (without Ciprofloxacin): **12.0%**

*Add ofloxacin=$4,080.00
Add amikacin=$27,648.00
Add clofazimine=$71.00

KEY: NA = not available.

[a] Treatment costs based on median prices given in table 5-1. Costs are for an entire recommended treatment cycle. Estimates include drug costs only.

SOURCE: U.S. Department of Health and Human Services, Public Health Service, Centers for Disease Control and Prevention, Division of Tuberculosis Elimination, 1993.

State statutes authorize State and local health agencies to control TB and other communicable diseases. Most of these agencies, in turn, contract with local hospitals and clinics to provide TB services. It is widely held, though infrequently documented, that these public health services have generally not kept pace with health problems in recent years, resulting in part from dwindling funds, lack of expertise, and outdated technologies. In addition, long waiting times, an inhospitable environment for personal care, and lack of flexible service hours in many public health clinics may also contribute to inadequate treatment.

As many specialized TB facilities closed during the 1960s and 1970s, much of the job of TB diagnosis and treatment has shifted to private primary care physicians, many of whom are unaccustomed to seeing patients with active TB or MDR-TB. These physicians may be less likely to suspect TB, diagnose it quickly, and prescribe the most efficacious treatment regimen. Recently collected data suggest that as many as 40 percent of physicians would unknowingly prescribe an inappropriate TB regimen, an error which could lead to treatment failure and emergence of drug resistance.

Even when an optimal drug regimen is prescribed, available, and feasible, patients do not always complete treatment. A very small percentage of patients do refuse or are mentally unable to follow treatment. Still, available evidence suggests that most patients would complete treatment if it were feasible to do so or if encouraged to do so through incentives and progressively more stringent measures as allowed by law to protect the public health.

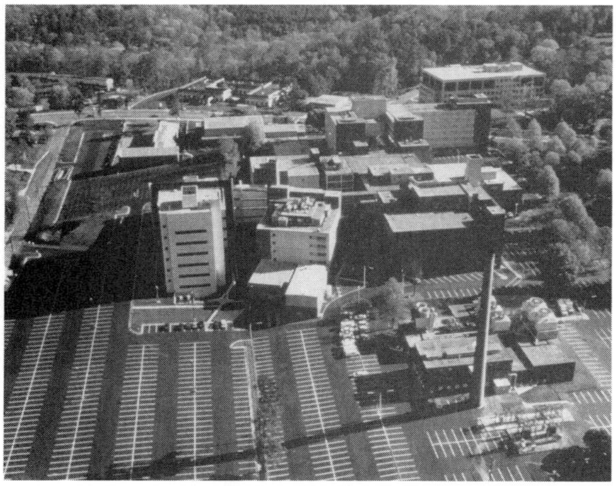

CENTERS FOR DISEASE CONTROL AND PREVENTION

The Centers for Disease Control and Prevention, headquartered in Altanta, has primary responsibility within the Federal Government for TB control.

A central issue in treatment delivery concerns the degree to which supervision by HCWs is necessary to bring about higher rates of treatment completion. One form of supervised treatment is directly observed treatment (DOT), which CDC defines as observation of the patient by a health care provider or other responsible person who has frequent contact with the patient as the patient ingests anti-TB medications. Although the concept of DOT is often proposed in policy and clinical discussions, often as an alternative to more restrictive forms of ensuring treatment completion, DOT can take many forms. Some programs limit DOT to health care facilities, while others send workers to patients' homes or other places. All DOT programs are labor-intensive and require skill, diligence, perseverance, and funds.

While some groups, including CDC and ALA, have recommended DOT be considered for every patient, others have argued that its use for most patients is wasteful and needlessly restrictive since they would complete therapy anyway. Most of the existing literature of different treatment delivery strategies are only descriptive in nature. ***Little systematic research has been done on the effectiveness or cost effectiveness of individual DOT strategies or of DOT compared to less supervised treatment for different patient populations. A more complete assessment of costs and outcomes is needed to generate useful information for public policy.***

Federal Involvement in TB Control

Primary responsibility for designing and carrying out TB control services rests with State and local health departments, not the Federal Government. Still, the Federal Government does provide the major funding, other resources, leadership, and coordination to the Nation's TB control efforts through several agencies. Only a few of these agencies are able to estimate spending for TB as distinct from funds for other responsibilities.

Public Health Activities

The Centers for Disease Control and Prevention make up the lead Federal agency for TB control. Out of its $79 million TB budget for fiscal year 1993, CDC gave $34.3 million in grants to State and local health departments. Another $39.2 million constituted emergency funds that Congress separately appropriated for TB control in six States and seven cities most heavily affected by TB. The remaining $5.2 million supported TB program operations at CDC itself. CDC also used $25.4 million designated for HIV activities for HIV-related TB efforts. Table 1-2 breaks down CDC's TB spending for fiscal year 1993 by function. These appropriations represented a major increase in TB funds over previous years (see figure 1-2). In addition, the President's fiscal year 1994 budget request includes $50 million over fiscal year 1993.

Following a drastic scaleback in Federal TB funding in the 1960s and 1970s, CDC restarted many of its activities in the early 1980s and developed a comprehensive ''Strategic Plan for the Elimination of Tuberculosis in the United States'' with the goal of lowering the incidence to 3.5 per 100,000 by the year 2000 and 0.1 per

Table 1-2—U.S. Centers for Disease Control and Prevention Spending for Tuberculosis by Function, Fiscal Year 1993

	Dollars ($ millions)	Percent of budget
Community-based control programs (screening, treatment, prevention, infection control)	$ 36.9	35%
Outreach and service linkage (implementation of directly observed therapy)	36.7	35
Research and demonstration	9.8	9
Surveillance, epidemiology and data systems	7.0	7
Laboratory services	4.8	5
Public education and information	4.4	4
Professional competence assurance (training for service providers, physicians, researchers, and laboratory personnel)	2.2	2
Leadership and administration (technical assistance to improve management of State and local TB control programs)	2.2	2
Community protection/regulatory programs	NA	NA
Total	$104.0	100%[a]

NA = not available.

[a] Component percentages do not add up to 100 percent due to rounding error.

SOURCE: Office of Technology Assessment, 1993, based on data from C. Bozzi, Assistant to the Director for Tuberculosis Coordination, Division of Tuberculosis Elimination, Public Health Service, Centers for Disease Control and Prevention, U.S. Department of Health and Human Services, Atlanta, GA, personal communication, July 9, 1993.

Figure 1-2—Tuberculosis Funding, U.S. Centers for Disease Control and Prevention, Fiscal Years 1960-93

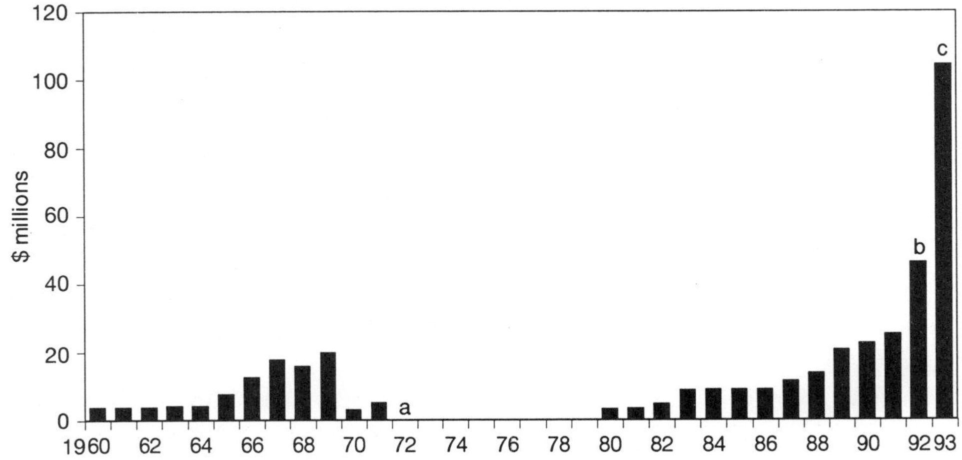

[a] Fiscal years 1972 through 1982 categorical grants ceased, funds to states were in block grants not specific for TB.

[b] Fiscal year 1992 includes $26 million in human immunodeficiency virus (HIV) funds, used for HIV-related TB activities.

[c] Fiscal year 1993 includes $25 million in HIV funds used for HIV-related TB activities.

SOURCE: Office of Technology Assessment, 1993, based on data from the U.S. Centers for Disease Control.

100,000 by 2010. In 1992, CDC headed a task force of Federal agencies and other public health groups that issued a complementary "National Action Plan to Combat MDR-TB." The task force plan, which targets all forms of TB, not just drug-resistant forms, details an exhaustive array of government and private responsibilities in TB control and research.

CDC estimates that Congress would need to increase CDC's budget for TB control by $380 million for fiscal year 1994 to implement fully CDC's responsibilities under the MDR-TB Action Plan. This amount is $330 million more than the amount actually requested in the President's 1994 budget. Estimates of money necessary for other agencies to implement their responsibilities under the action plan are not currently available.

Other Federal agencies run health care facilities that provide TB treatment. These agencies include the Department of Veterans Affairs, the Indian Health Service, and the Federal Bureau of Prisons. In addition to supporting some anti-TB drug research and the development of educational materials on TB for health professionals, the Department of Health and Human Services' (U.S. DHHS) Health Resources and Services Administration (HRSA) funds TB services through State and locally run clinics that serve disadvantaged and underserved populations. The U.S. Agency for International Development (U.S. AID) gave over $8 million for TB control in developing countries, most of which supported BCG vaccination of children. Other agencies with roles in TB control include the U.S. DHHS Substance Abuse and Mental Services Administration (SAMHSA), Department of State's consular offices and embassies abroad, the Department of Justice's Immigration and Naturalization Service (INS), and the Department of Labor's Occupational Safety and Health Administration (OSHA).

Research and Development

Most Federal TB-related research and development (R&D) is conducted or funded by the National Institutes of Health (NIH). Its spending for TB research has increased dramatically from $4.2 million in fiscal year 1991 to $35.9 million in fiscal year 1993, with an additional $10 million requested by the President in his fiscal year 1994 budget proposal.[8] The bulk of NIH's funding (57 percent) for fiscal year 1993 is administered by the National Institute of Allergy and Infectious Disease (NIAID), although a total of 17 NIH institutes and centers within NIH report ongoing TB research.

NIAID estimates that full funding of those activities in the MDR-TB National Action Plan that fall within NIAID's purview would cost $45.6 million in fiscal year 1994, $20.6 million above NIAID's spending in fiscal year 1993. In spring 1993, an NIH Executive Committee identified and prioritized new TB research opportunities for all of NIH. Fully funding this research agenda would cost an estimated $102 million above fiscal year 1993 funding.

Areas of NIH research include development of new diagnostic tools, drugs, and vaccines as well as behavioral issues on prevention of transmission and adherence to treatment. NIH is also spending $2.3 million to convert an existing building into a containment laboratory that allows for the safe handling of drug-resistant strains of tubercle bacilli. Too few containment laboratories at NIH and other research institutions limit the amount of TB research scientists can conduct (29,30).

The Office of Technology Assessment (OTA) found a lack of systematic research on the effectiveness or cost-effectiveness of individual interventions to control TB infection in hospitals or to ensure that patients in different communities or treatment settings complete anti-TB therapy. In addition, little effort in health services and health

---

[8] The 1993 budget includes $14.1 million also counted as HIV spending and $4.8 in one-time funds transferred by the NIH director from her discretionary budget.

economics research has been devoted to understanding variation in the use of hospitalization and costs of treating TB, especially during the disease's acute, infectious period.

Although CDC and some institutes at NIH are conducting studies on the effectiveness and appropriateness of TB services, U.S. DHHS's Agency for Health Care Policy and Research (AHCPR) takes the lead in conducting and supporting federally sponsored health services, health economics, and medical care effectiveness research. AHCPR's main efforts so far on TB were its participation in developing the MDR-TB National Action Plan and a 1993 workshop for judges on HIV and TB.

Regulation of TB Technology

The Food and Drug Administration ensures the safety and effectiveness of drugs used to treat TB. It also regulates and approves BCG and other vaccines, tuberculin skin tests, other diagnostic reagents used to detect *M.tb.* or to determine drug susceptibility, and devices used to prevent the spread of the disease. In recent years, FDA's role in TB control has focused on alleviating shortages of some TB drugs and expediting the approval of new TB drugs. The FDA recently helped make available an interim supply of SM and PAS for MDR-TB patients through CDC when adequate amounts of the drug could not be obtained privately. The FDA is also working with companies to encourage development of combination drugs and new technologies such as implantable, slow-release formulations.

Federal Disability Programs

The Social Security Administration (SSA) administers two programs for people unable to work due to disability—the Disability Insurance (DI) program for those who have paid the requisite social security taxes over the course of their careers, and the Supplemental Security Income (SSI) program for very low-income individuals. While SSI pays a set amount each month and can begin once the beneficiary is forced to stop work, DI benefits depend on the amount of social security taxes paid by the beneficiary; DI has a 5-month waiting period after the onset of disability.

By law, both programs require that an applicant be unable to work due to a physical or mental impairment expected to result in death or to last at least a year. SSI and DI are not available for most patients with drug-susceptible TB because they are usually able to work once a few weeks of treatment renders them noncontagious. However, TB patients can qualify for SSI or DI if they also have concurrent HIV or if they have some other disabling condition.

Medicaid and Medicare

While many medical services for people with active TB are provided directly in outpatient clinics through State and local programs that do not necessarily charge patients, third-party health insurers also pay for some TB services for their beneficiaries. Little if any systematic research has been done on the role of insurance in financing care for TB. However, indirect evidence does suggest a significant role for Federal insurance programs. Figure 1-3, which breaks down all hospitalizations for TB in 16 States in 1990 according to payer, shows that Medicaid was the single most likely payer (36 percent), with Medicare paying for another 17 percent. In total, government pays for almost three-quarters of TB hospitalizations in these States.[9]

Medicaid, a State-administered program funded jointly by the Federal and State governments, provides health insurance to certain categories of low-income individuals, including recipients of SSI, many poor women and children, and, in some States, people whose high medical bills make them poor or almost poor. The minimum set of

[9] Although not necessarily representative of the entire country, the States presented do include several with the highest TB burdens, most notably New York and California.

Figure 1-3—Hospital Admissions With a Diagnosis of Tuberculosis in 16 States[a] by Payer, 1990

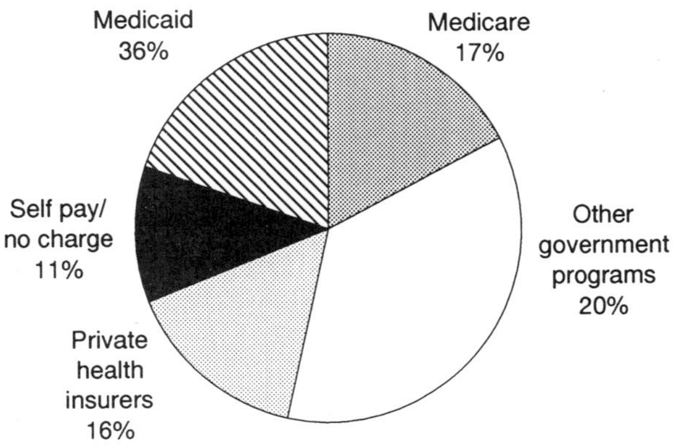

[a] States are Arizona, California, Colorado, Florida, Massachusetts, Maine, New Hampshire, New Jersey, Nevada, New York, Oregon, Pennsylvania, South Carolina, Vermont, Washington, and Wisconsin.

SOURCE: Office of Technology Assessment, 1993 based on data derived from State hospital discharge abstracts covering 100 percent of acute short-stay hospitals and U.S. Department of Veterans Affairs hospitals. Data prepared by Codman Research Group, Inc., Lebanon, New Hampshire.

benefits provided under Medicaid covers inpatient, outpatient, laboratory, and other services for TB patients at approved facilities.

With approval from the Federal Health Care Financing Administration (HCFA) that administers Medicaid and Medicare, New York's Medicaid program pays for directly observed therapy for Medicaid-eligible TB patients with reimbursement amounts dependent on the intensity of effort necessary to provide and supervise therapy. No other State has yet attempted innovative approaches to providing TB services with Medicaid funding. HCFA estimates that in 1991, the Federal Government's portion of Medicaid spending for TB totaled $45 million, while the States' portion totaled $30 million.

Medicare provides health insurance to individuals who are over age 65, who have end-stage renal disease, or who have received Social Security DI benefits for 2 years. Medicare pays for inpatient services provided in short-stay hospitals and ambulatory services provided in an office or clinic under a physician's supervision. Although Medicare does contain some limited home health care benefits and long-term care and skilled nursing services in certain types of approved facilities, DOT in the home and long-term care facilities dedicated to TB care would most likely not qualify for Medicare reimbursement. HCFA estimates that Medicare spending for TB totaled $65 million in 1991.

Policy Options for Congress

Through its analysis, OTA has identified 11 options for congressional consideration (box 1-A). Each option has the underlying goal of improving TB control capabilities in the United States. They fall into three categories that affect:

- The public health infrastructure for combating TB;
- The research, development, and availability of technologies for combating TB; and
- The financial security and financial access to health care services for persons with, or at risk of, TB.

The focus of this discussion is on potential actions of the Federal Government in providing leadership and resources for the Nation's TB control activities, rather than on potential actions of the State, local, and private authorities that carry out many of the programs to fight this disease. A fuller discussion of these options and their potential implications follows.

Options That Affect The Public Health Infrastructure for Combating TB

OPTION 1. *Fully fund the public health activities identified in the CDC's 1992 National Action Plan to Combat Multidrug-Resistant Tuberculosis.*

CDC estimates that full implementation of all activities in its 1992 National Action Plan to combat MDR-TB (described in box 7-B) for which it would be responsible would require appropriations of $380 million during the first year over and above the $105 million appropriated in fiscal year 1993. This estimate includes

Box 1-A—Policy Options for Congressional Consideration

Option 1. Fund fully the public health activities identified in the CDC's 1992 National Action Plan to Combat Multidrug-Resistant Tuberculosis.

Option 2. Establish a mechanism for direct Federal intervention in cities and other jurisdictions with extraordinarily high levels of active tuberculosis, multidrug-resistant TB, or HIV and TB coinfection.

Option 3. Require universal directly observed treatment (DOT) through legislation, regulation, or as a condition of receiving Federal TB control funds.

Option 4. Require periodic TB skin testing, active case finding (by chest x-ray), and preventive treatment in Federal hospitals, prisons, and other facilities.

Option 5. Purchase directly anti-TB drugs and distribute them to State and local authorities.

Option 5a. Purchase directly anti-TB drugs with State and local authorities reimbursing the Federal Government.

Option 6. Increase support for international TB control activities.

Option 7. Make a concerted effort to develop health services research relevant to the fight against TB.

Option 8. Fully fund basic and clinical TB research as outlined in the CDC's 1992 National Action Plan to Combat Multidrug-Resistant Tuberculosis and NIH's 1993 Tuberculosis Research Opportunities.

Option 9. Support the creation of additional regional "centers of excellence" for TB treatment and research.

Option 10. Expand the Federal Government's definition of disability to include active TB as a disabling condition for the purposes of Supplemental Security Income (SSI) and Disability Insurance (DI) benefits.

Option 11. Provide States with the option to expand categorical Medicaid coverage to persons without other forms of health insurance who have tuberculous infection or active TB.

Option 11a. Limit the option of expanding categorical Medicaid eligibility to those with active disease only.

Option 11b. Limit categorical Medicaid eligibility to TB-related services only.

SOURCE: Office of Technology Assessment, 1993.

$62 million in R&D expenditures, with the remainder allocated toward various forms of public health activities. Although CDC currently has no estimates of amounts that would be required for subsequent years, the $380 million increase would include some one-year-only spending as well as some spending that would be continued subsequently (35). No estimates currently exist of the cost of fully implementing activities in the National Action Plan that are the responsibility of other Federal agencies.

OTA found that CDC and other TB experts agreed on the need for increased Federal involvement and resources. However, some of the options that follow in this section highlight major policy questions that would need answers to fully implement the CDC plan. In addition, because CDC has given only rough indicators of priority among all of the actions it recommends, Congress and other policymakers cannot evaluate in detail how CDC and other Federal agencies would propose to allocate funding increases if Congress appropriated less than the amount required for full implementation.

Immediate full funding of the plan may not be more effective or more efficient than a more incremental phase-in. On the one hand, such a dramatic increase in funding would alert the country to the threat of TB to affected communities and the value the Federal Government places on TB control.

On the other hand, the public health and research system may not be able to absorb such a large influx of cash as efficiently as it could if the increases came more gradually. In the course of OTA's analysis, public health officials pointed out the highly regulated and slow process some State and local governments face in hiring qualified individuals to administer TB therapy and to perform other public health functions (29,30). Additional Federal grants would not immediately increase the supply of qualified public health workers or speed up local governmental hiring processes. Also, this report highlights the lack of information about the relative effectiveness of individual infection control procedures. Without first developing better experimental data on these technologies,[10] some money devoted to retrofitting hospital rooms and other facilities to serve active TB patients would probably be spent inefficiently or unnecessarily. In an era of limited Federal resources and many competing public health needs, policymakers may wish to weigh the value for spending some TB control dollars better in the future against the value of providing maximum resources for TB now.

OPTION 2. *Establish a mechanism for direct Federal intervention in cities and other jurisdictions with extraordinarily high levels of active TB, MDR-TB, or HIV and TB coinfection.*

Support for this option would rest on the assumption that TB can pose a significant enough threat in some communities that State and local authorities alone are unable to respond quickly and sufficiently, even with Federal financial support. One TB expert suggested to OTA that the magnitude of drug resistance, HIV dual infection, substance abuse, homelessness, and incomplete TB treatment is great enough in New York City to warrant the formation of a Federal task force to supply personnel and expertise from elsewhere on a short-term, emergency basis (29,30).[11] Such a plan would extend the technical expertise that CDC routinely provides to State and local health authorities. Federal personnel would help provide TB treatment, find cases of TB in facilities that public health officials suspect to harbor the disease, and perform other TB services needed in the community.

This option raises several questions. First, by what criteria would the Federal Government decide to intervene? Given that most legal authority to protect the public health has been traditionally vested in State and local governments (125), any Federal intervention would almost certainly, at a minimum, require a request from the relevant local governments. Second, Federal officials would need to develop epidemiologic or other criteria for judging that TB has reached levels high enough to justify this Federal action. These criteria would need to be measurable and perhaps flexible. Inclusion of TB and HIV coinfection rates or numbers of foreign-born residents, if measurable, could make this option available for communities with low rates of existing TB but the potential for high rates in the future. The emphasis of Federal intervention in these communities may be on screening high-risk groups and preventive treatment, rather than on providing resources for treating active disease.

Decisionmakers would also want to question whether Federal Government intervention would actually be more effective than the local governments and private organizations acting alone. As noted, the ability to bring in Federal personnel

[10] The initiation of such research is itself included in the Action Plan.

[11] This suggestion was not made by an official of the New York State or City governments.

may offer a significant advantage for State and local governments that face limitations in hiring, although the Federal Government may also face hiring restrictions. Reassignment of professionals from the Commissioned Public Health Service Corps would mean these individuals would be unable to continue to fulfill their current responsibilities.

The cost of hiring additional Federal personnel on a short-term basis would depend on the number hired, their qualifications, the duration of their employment, and perhaps whether they currently reside in the targeted community or must relocate. Another possibility would be to make voluntary service on such task forces one means of paying back government loans for health professional education and training as was done in greater numbers during the 1970s and 1980s under the National Health Service Corps. There is also precedent for providing special visas for qualified foreign medical personnel to fill positions in underserved areas.

OPTION 3. *Require universal directly observed treatment (DOT) through legislation, regulation, or as a condition of receiving Federal TB control funds.*

The American Lung Association recently recommended DOT for all persons with active TB (244). In contrast, CDC has recommended that DOT be considered for active cases.

Supporters of universal DOT point to the practical difficulty of predicting *a priori* which patients will complete treatment without supervision. These supporters argue that human nature should lead health professionals to expect that patients will forget to take medication without reminders. Universal DOT proponents also argue that some health authorities may be more likely to assume that homeless individuals, drug users, and people without access to regular health care would be less likely than other TB patients to complete therapy. These groups may be subjected to more restrictive treatment measures without a strong medical or public health rationale. Requiring universal DOT helps insure that all TB patients are treated in an equitable manner.

Opponents of requiring universal DOT point out that despite the difficulties in predicting who is unlikely to complete treatment, between 1976 and 1990, over 80 percent of persons with active TB in the United States completed treatment without DOT (9). One estimate for New York City suggests that DOT costs may fall between $2,000 and $3,000 per person excluding the cost of drugs (29,30). Opponents argue that universal DOT is a wasteful use of limited resources and needlessly intrusive for most patients.

In addition, Federal policymakers would need to define exactly what State and local governments would have to do to conform to the Federal requirement. DOT can take many different forms and degrees of restrictiveness, require varying intensities of resources, and be combined with a variety of complementary programs such as incentives or inducements to complete therapy.

As suggested in chapter 6, there are more options available to policymakers than just requiring DOT for everybody or trying to predict *a priori* which TB patients will not complete therapy. One alternative, used in some communities, is to monitor all patients' therapy, but allow their behaviors to be indicators of the need for more intensive supervision of therapy. Only when patients do not show up for medical appointments or give other evidence that they might not complete therapy would public health officials require patients to be observed taking their medications. Although this alternative to universal DOT requires that public health authorities have the resources to track down missing patients quickly, a potentially difficult and labor-intensive task, particularly for homeless or other difficult-to-locate patients, it may be less expensive and as effective in some communities.

OPTION 4. *Require periodic TB skin testing, active case finding (by chest x-ray) and preventive treatment in Federal hospitals, prisons, and other facilities.*

Epidemiological evidence indicates that hospitals, prisons, and other facilities housing people in congregate settings may be appropriate targets for TB prevention because institutions house many individuals at high risk of progressing to active disease. Identifying infected residents and workers at high risk of developing active TB, as well as those who already have active TB, offers an opportunity to prevent the potential spread of the disease to others with whom the active cases have close contact. Immigrants, currently screened for active disease for legal entry into the United States, are another high-risk group that the Federal Government may wish to consider for screening and preventive treatment if found to have tuberculous infection.

Positive skin tests would help identify candidates for preventive treatment, although health officials would have to consider the problem of false negative among immunocompromised individuals with tuberculous infection. In addition, officials would need to consider the best way to use chest x-ray technology in order to identify active disease.

By requiring screening and preventive treatment programs in its own facilities, the Federal Government would be setting a standard that could encourage State and local authorities to adopt voluntarily for their own congregate institutions. However, there are some potential drawbacks to a Federal policy. The Federal agencies charged with administering each type of institution may not correctly identify groups at high enough risk of active disease to warrant screening and follow-up preventive treatment.

For example, many patients admitted to Veterans Administration or other Federal hospitals for short periods of time may be at very low risk of developing active TB if infected. In addition, nonfederal institutions attempting to follow the Federal Government's lead might also establish screening programs where they are likely to yield little benefit. Workplace screening in low-risk settings such as a factory are unlikely to have much effect on the spread of much TB. Analysis in this report suggests that research into the most cost-effective ways of running screening and preventive treatment programs may not be available to guide the implementation of this option.

Funding for screening and prevention in Federal institutions would presumably come from the budgets of the agencies charged with administering them as do most current TB control efforts. The Department of Veterans Affairs (U.S. DVA) currently pays for TB control in its own hospitals, the Bureau of Prisons in Federal prisons, and so on. This decentralized administration of Federal facilities raises the further problem of ensuring compliance with a screening and prevention requirement. Current Bureau of Prisons policy already requires chest x-rays for new inmates and tuberculin skin testing every 2 years, but no data are available on the extent to which such testing is actually carried out. Adoption of screening requirements would require mechanisms to ensure they are carried out as well as sufficient resources to ensure appropriate diagnostic followup and treatment; this includes not just money, but trained personnel as well.

OPTION 5. *Directly purchase anti-TB drugs and distribute them to State and local authorities.*

The rationale behind universal TB drug purchase is that the Federal Government, acting as a single, large-volume buyer should get the needed pharmaceuticals at a lower cost than can individual States or local health departments. The same considerations could apply to universal purchase of PPD skin testing kits.

The Federal Government already purchases some childhood vaccines under contract at prices substantially below retail. The CDC's recent survey of trends in anti-TB drug prices revealed that the price paid for the same form and dose of a drug can vary greatly from State to State. In addition, if the Federal Government were to take on the function of paying for all TB drugs, State and local governments could use the money that would have gone to pharmaceutical purchase for other purposes.

CDC currently has the statutory authority to take on this activity; it requires only the appropriations to do so. CDC estimates that in 1993, the cost of purchasing all anti-TB drugs used at the State and local levels would total $80 million. This figure is included in the CDC's estimates of fully implementing its National Action Plan for the elimination of TB.

However, this amount of money would cover only the cost of the drugs themselves and does not include the cost of administering the drug purchase program or distributing the pharmaceuticals. CDC currently has no estimates of the costs of these functions. It is also not clear whether the Federal Government would take on the function of distributing the drugs to the States or whether that function would continue to be done by the drug suppliers. U.S. DVA currently purchases drugs in bulk for use in its own hospitals, but does so with a highly centralized distribution system, thus minimizing the distribution costs borne by the pharmaceutical suppliers. The willingness of suppliers to give discounts for bulk purchasing may be partially dependent on whether the Federal Government took on responsibility for distributing the drugs since the suppliers' costs would be lower.

CDC has not indicated the assumptions that went into its $80 million estimate. Not only is it not clear what prices the government would expect to pay for each pharmaceutical, but also CDC has not shown how improved case finding might increase drug costs in subsequent years or how decreases in TB rates would ultimately decrease funds necessary to purchase drugs.

The final price negotiated for these drugs could also depend on the number of manufacturers for a drug. Some of the more expensive drugs are still covered by patents and hence only have one manufacturer. When manufacturers do not face competition, they may not see an incentive to give significant discounts in order to sell their products. In other cases, there may be only one manufacturer of a drug or its active ingredient even though it is no longer covered by a patent (121,152). These manufacturers may also be reluctant to give significant discounts. Finally, the pharmaceutical industry has suggested that centralized purchase would provide an added disincentive for firms to invest in research to develop new drugs as discussed in option 8 below (286).

OPTION 5a. *Directly purchase anti-TB drugs with State and local authorities reimbursing the Federal Government.*

This option would be identical to Option 5 except that the Federal Government would not bear the $80 million estimated to be necessary for the purchase of the pharmaceuticals themselves. Instead, State and local governments would continue to pay for drugs, but would reap any cost savings the Federal Government can realize by purchasing on their behalf. Such cost savings might not be spread evenly among the States. The CDC survey indicates that some States, presumably those purchasing large quantities of drugs, already receive a discount through negotiated contracts with drug suppliers. These States would likely benefit less per unit of drug purchased than would areas of the country paying higher retail prices for their TB drugs.

OPTION 6. *Increase support for international TB control activities.*

The American Lung Association, among others, advocates greater support of the World Health Organization's TB programs, greater CDC provision of its technical staff to international organizations, and selected nations, more support for TB research in developing countries through NIH, and greater involvement of AID in tuberculosis control as well as in bilateral programs with other countries and through WHO (85). As noted in chapter 7, the Federal Government supports each of these activities to a certain extent, although the vast bulk of current and expected TB spending is targeted to the United States.

If Congress decided to increase TB control efforts in less developed countries, it could decide to do so purely on humanitarian grounds. However, even if Congress sought only to protect this nation's health, controlling TB abroad could lower TB incidence of the disease here given the mobility of foreign born people to the United States. Research oriented toward developing countries could also have benefits at home; for example, a fast, definitive diagnostic test designed for developing countries that do not have easy access to sophisticated clinical laboratories could be of great use in many urban and rural areas of the United States as well.

A potential danger of increasing United States support of TB efforts abroad is that it might divert resources from domestic TB control activities. The Federal Government has already laid out an ambitious domestic agenda to control TB for which there may not be sufficient funds to fully implement in the short-run. If money for expanded TB control efforts outside the United States would come from appropriations that would otherwise go to domestic public health and research activities, Congress may need to weigh the value of supporting efforts abroad against the impact that money would have on the health of people with TB at home.

Options That Affect the Research, Development, and Availability of Technologies for Combating TB

OPTION 7. *Make a concerted effort to develop health services research relevant to the fight against tuberculosis and to disseminate research results to policymakers and health professionals.*

Several areas of this report suggest that better health services and economic research results could help policymakers target TB control efforts more efficiently. Through legislation or through direction of U.S. DHHS, relevant agencies such as the CDC, AHCPR, HCFA, NIH, and HRSA could publicize TB health services research as a priority in various types of extramural funding programs. Several of these agencies have said they intend to expand their efforts in this area. Two sample questions suggested by OTA's analysis that might be answered by health services and health economics research are:

- What are the effectiveness and cost-effectiveness of various forms of DOT and how do these measures vary among different parts of the country and different groups of patients?
- What sources of income do TB patients have and what impact do government benefits have on the identification, treatment, and control of TB such as through SSI, Aid to Families with Dependent Children, housing programs, and food stamps?

This option could include efforts to disseminate to policymakers and health professionals the results of both health services and clinic research to improve the delivery of health services and to ensure appropriate clinical treatment for TB.

One drawback of this such research is that it could draw resources away from direct TB control. Data on the effectiveness and cost-effectiveness of treatment strategies such as DOT are best gained through randomized clinical trials, which are expensive. In addition, the size of such studies increases as one wants to learn more about differences in effectiveness among different sociodemographic groups or according to other ways that differentiate TB patients. Policymakers would also want to consider health services research already being undertaken by State and local governments and private groups such as foundations to assess its quality and to avoid duplication.

CDC's estimates of funds necessary to implement its responsibilities under the 1992 National Action Plan include funds for the health services and health economics it hopes to carry out. Estimates of funds needed for new health sources research that other Federal agencies would support are not available.

OPTION 8. *Fully fund basic and clinical TB research as outlined in the CDC's 1992 National Action Plan to Combat Multidrug-Resistant Tuberculosis and NIH's 1993 Tuberculosis Research Opportunities.*

CDC estimates that its research under the 1992 National Action Plan would cost $62 million in the first year above fiscal year 1993 spending. NIH estimates that new TB research would cost $102 million over several years. These research activities include not only basic research on the TB organism and its behavior in the human body, but also clinical investigations of new forms of prophylaxis, diagnosis, and treatment; the experimental study of environmental infection control technologies; and relevant human behavioral research.

On the rate of funding increases, the same considerations for policymakers described under Option 1 apply here. The ability of the scientific infrastructure to absorb funding for certain types of TB research include a limited number of researchers and clinicians trained to perform work in this area and a limited number of biomedical laboratories with sufficient containment facilities to prevent accidental infection of laboratory staff and others. On the other hand, some researchers have suggested that increases in funding will naturally lead to an increased capacity to do research (152).

As with Option 1, clarification of funding priorities for R&D activities would help Congress and other policymakers understand better the implications of partial or phased-in funding of the CDC National Action Plan. NIH has provided detailed priorities for research projects in its plan. In addition, analysis in this report suggests several areas of relatively high priority: development of faster and definitive diagnostic and drug susceptibility testing techniques, development of new anti-tuberculosis drugs, and the development of easier-to-use dosage forms of the treatments, such as combinations of commonly used drugs and slowly released, implantable formulations, and new research to bolster our understanding of the TB bacilli and its manifestations in the human body.

The area of drug development raises a few additional issues for the Federal Government. The FDA indicates that some drug companies have been reluctant to develop a drug for both TB and non-TB uses for fear that many physicians would reserve the drug for TB treatment only rather than using it for more common infections. The companies fear that these implicit restrictions of the drugs' use would limit the revenue they generate and their ability to recoup the manufacturers' initial R&D costs. In addition, the pharmaceutical industry is concerned about disincentives to engage in research should the Federal Government attempt to force discounts for TB drugs as discussed in Option 5 (120).[12]

This situation suggests that there are important constraints other than funding and resources in making new therapies available. Congress, executive branch agencies, and groups outside of government may wish to examine new ways to encourage drug industry participation in TB drug development beyond those that the FDA has already tried. New ideas could run the gamut of measures, from focusing public attention on the need for new treatments, to clarifying the applicability of orphan drug subsidies to this area,[13] and to offering new, more direct financial incentives.

OPTION 9. *Support the creation of additional regional "centers of excellence" for TB treatment and research.*

Several centers that specialize in the treatment of drug-susceptible and more complicated cases

---

[12] The FDA cites the classes of drugs known as qunolones and macrolides as potential examples.

[13] To encourage the development of new treatments for conditions that affect fewer than 200,000 persons in the United States, the Orphan Drug Law (Public Law 97-414) provides incentives including a 7-year market exclusivity as well as grants and tax credits to support clinical research. Currently, active TB fits the definition of an orphan condition.

of TB already exist.[14] One TB expert has suggested establishing a total of 6 to 12 centers funded at a cost of about $5 million each per year (29,30). In addition to treating difficult cases and training TB clinicians and researchers who would pursue future work on this disease, these centers would provide an opportunity to study and disseminate new technologies for the diagnosis and treatment of TB. Not only would researchers be able to study the technologies under relatively controlled conditions, but also the centers could train clinicians and technicians in their use.

The main question for policymakers is whether establishing additional centers is the most efficient public policy to treat difficult patients, train TB professionals, and bring together TB research interests. Even if it were an efficient approach to TB care, research, and training, it is not clear whether 6 to 12 centers (or any other suggested number) are commensurate with the threat posed by TB. It is also not clear how sick patients would be before they would have to be transferred to the centers for treatment. Policymakers would want to consider the number of patients in need of such specialized services in determining how many centers the country needs. The existence of such centers might encourage their use for some patients that could be treated in institutions closer to their homes. Furthermore, once the current epidemic is brought under control, the country might not need as many such centers.

Policymakers may want to understand better whether there would be cost or other advantages to treating patients in centers instead of other institutions. They may also want to consider whether existing institutions could be modified for less than the cost of establishing a new center to conduct biomedical TB research. Similarly, it might be possible to train clinicians and other professionals sufficiently in existing institutions for less money.

Another issue that would need to be examined is how centers would be reimbursed for the care of patients from a separate jurisdiction if the cost of such care would usually be borne by the health department or Medicaid program where the patient currently usually lives. The centers would also require trained personnel who may only be available in sufficient numbers over time.

Options That Affect the Financial Security and Financial Access to Housing and Health Care Services for Persons with or at Risk of TB

OPTION 10. *Expand the Federal Government's definition of disability to include active TB as a disabling condition for the purposes of Supplemental Security Income and Disability Insurance benefits.*

Underlying this proposal is the observation that many people with active TB are in precarious financial situations. Their poverty may interfere with their ability to receive treatment and to prevent transmission of the disease to others. Many TB patients are homeless. For disabled individuals without other sources of income, SSI provides a very basic subsistence and categorical eligibility for Medicaid health insurance. In the case of substance abusers, many residential treatment programs have been successful in receiving SSI to cover some of the costs of those patients in treatment may last more than a year.

As described in Chapter 7, most individuals with TB alone are not considered disabled because their condition does not prevent them from working for a year or longer. Changing this rule in order to make active TB patients eligible for SSI would require congressional legislation to amend the Social Security Act. In passing such legislation, Congress would also need to decide whether this exception applies only to the SSI program or whether it would also apply to the DI

[14] These include National Jewish Hospital in Denver, Colorado, the University of Medicine and Dentistry of New Jersey in Newark, New Jersey and Bellevue Hospital in New York City.

program as well since both currently rely on the same definition and processes for determining disability.

A new law would establish a significant exception to one of the most basic tenets of current disability policy. A major drawback of this option is that it would use a disability program to provide financial benefits to a group of people who are not disabled according to the way Congress has defined disability over the history of the SSI and DI programs. In adopting this option, Congress could be opening a Pandora's box of requests to use disability programs as a means of providing income to other groups of individuals who are not currently considered disabled.

A proposal to revise the SSA's disability definition to include TB may reflect two other problems perceived by proponents of this option: 1) a perceived lack of coordination of all public benefits for which TB patients may currently be eligible, and 2) a lack of resources to provide housing for many TB patients in some areas of the country.

To the extent these two perceived problems are real, the Federal Government, along with State and local authorities, may wish to consider other options for coordination of relevant Federal benefits for each case of active TB and directly to consider other ways the Federal Government could help alleviate TB patients' need for housing. Dealing with these policy problems directly may be preferable to setting a precedent of using disability programs in ways they were not designed. Specific actions to provide housing are not included in the CDC's 1992 National Action Plan.

One alternative action for policymakers that would not require a change in statute would be to educate patients and their caregivers to make sure TB patients currently eligible for SSI already because of HIV, substance abuse, or protracted TB treatment actually apply for the program.

OPTION 11. *Provide States with the option to expand categorical Medicaid coverage to persons without other forms of health insurance who have tuberculous infection or active TB.*

Over the years, Congress has expanded categorical Medicaid eligibility, especially for certain groups of women and children. Congress offers States the option of extending eligibility to all persons with tuberculous infection or active disease with the usual mix of Federal and State funds. The added cost of this option to State or Federal Medicaid budgets is uncertain. For the State government, the cost largely depends on the prevalence of TB in the State. For the Federal Government, it depends on how many and which States decide to adopt the option. In addition, to the extent that patients with TB have other medical problems but were not previously covered by Medicaid, the costs of expanding Medicaid eligibility would be more than just those costs associated with TB care.

This option would transfer some share of the burden for TB services from public health department budgets to the Medicaid program at both the Federal and State levels. The option would also reinforce the trend toward the "privatization" of TB services (noted in chapter 6), shifting the focus of TB control from public health activities to individual, reimbursable health services. Another impact of this option would be to add to the administrative costs of State Medicaid programs in processing applications for eligibility and claims reimbursement. Finally, as noted in chapter 6, financial access is not the only factor in ensuring that patients receive and complete treatment; expanding Medicaid eligibility does not guarantee that there will be enough trained professionals to provide and supervise appropriate therapy.

OPTION 11a. *Limit the option of expanding categorical Medicaid eligibility to those with active disease only.*

Although limiting Medicaid coverage to active disease cases only would reduce the cost of this option, it would also exclude from Medicaid reimbursement any diagnostic services and preventive therapy for people with tuberculous infection (unless the infected patients were eligible for Medicaid through some other provision in the Medicaid statutes).

OPTION 11b. *Limit categorical Medicaid eligibility to TB-related services only.*

This option would also save money by limiting the reimbursement to services related to TB only. Under this option, Congress could cover all people with tuberculous infection or limit coverage to those with active TB only.[15] This option has the disadvantage of excluding treatments for other conditions the individual may have, such as HIV. Treatment for these other conditions not only affects the individual's overall health, but can affect his or her ability to recover from TB itself. However, some portion of patients with both TB and other conditions like HIV would qualify for full Medicaid eligibility through other provisions in the Medicaid statutes.

[15] While this report was in its final publishing stages, Congress adopted a version of this option (P.L.103-66) giving States the opportunity to use Medicaid funds to pay for TB services only for low income individuals with either tuberculous infection or active disease who do not otherwise qualify for Medicaid.

Etiology and Transmission of Tuberculosis | 2

Tuberculosis (TB) was once commonly called "consumption" because of the wasting patients suffered. Its former medical name "phthisis" also referred to the progressive wasting or consumptive condition of patients with the disease. Its current name refers instead to a histological feature of the disease: the characteristic presence of nodular lesions, or "tubercles," in the early stages of the disease.

The infectious nature of TB and the agent responsible for its transmission from person to person have been known for over a hundred years: in 1882, the German scientist Robert Koch identified a species of bacteria, *Mycobacterium tuberculosis* (*M.tb.* or tubercle bacilli), as the cause of TB (169).[1] Despite this single underlying cause, clinical manifestations of the disease vary from person to person and the ways in which the body controls the infection or allows it to progress to a destructive disease state are still not adequately understood. Furthermore, concurrent human immunodeficiency virus (HIV) infection appears to impair some of the critical immune processes involved in preventing tuberculous infection from progressing to disease, creating a somewhat different clinical course for individuals who are dually infected. Infants and young children generally manifest tuberculous infection and disease differently from adults, but have many of the characteristics of TB in HIV-infected adults.

This chapter provides background information about TB transmission and disease processes relevant to topics covered in

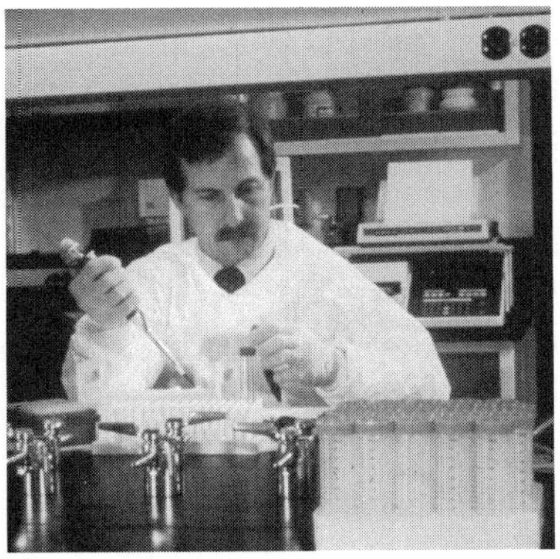

[1] Other types of mycobacteria can cause tuberculosis in humans, but are not significant contributors to the disease in the United States. Earlier this century, *M. bovis*, which causes TB in cattle, was transmitted to human beings through unpasteurized milk and respiratory exposure to infected cattle, but now accounts for less than 1 percent of human TB cases in North America (347).

other chapters of this report. The factors involved in transmitting tuberculous infection and in developing active disease are summarized first, followed by a brief description of the clinical course of the disease in immunocompetent and immunocompromised individuals and in children.

TRANSMISSION AND INFECTIVITY

TB has two general stages relevant to its transmission and infectivity: **tuberculous infection** (sometimes also called "latent TB") and **active tuberculosis.** As used in this report and in most of the medical literature, TB refers primarily to the active disease. Although infection with tubercle bacilli is necessary to develop TB, the majority (90 percent) of immunocompetent adults with tuberculous infection do not develop TB. The only evidence of their infection may be a positive tuberculin skin test (see chapter 4). Children and immunocompromised individuals with tuberculous infection carry a greater risk for developing active TB (see below).

Individuals with tuberculous infection are asymptomatic and not contagious to others, whereas individuals with active pulmonary disease may be symptomatic and contagious—particularly if they are untreated or inadequately treated and if the disease is manifested in the lungs (or, rarely, in the larynx). Regarding risk of transmission, the critical difference between the two types is the ability to expel (e.g., through coughing, singing, speaking, or sneezing) airborne particles containing viable tubercle bacilli.

As airborne infections go, TB is not considered the most contagious; certain airborne viral infections, such as measles and varicella (chicken pox), are more readily transmitted (66,204). However, because TB can be transmitted through casual contact (breathing) and it can be debilitating or even fatal if untreated (or untreatable, as in some cases of multidrug-resistant TB (MDR-TB)), the public's perception of the actual risk of TB contagion has generally been magnified. Health departments and TB centers report increased demand for tuberculin skin testing among very low risk individuals or the "worried-well" (129,243). A recent editorial in the *Washington Post* described TB as a highly contagious, deadly disease that "you can catch from the person next to you in a movie theater or classroom" (49).

According to available data, both from decades ago and the present, a single, casual contact with an infectious person in a public place (such as a subway or movie theater) is unlikely to lead to tuberculous infection, although the risk is not zero; there is a possibility, albeit remote, that inhalation of just one infectious particle containing *M.tb.* could be enough to produce infection in some cases (31). In practical terms, however, much more than a single airborne bacillus is needed to cause infection. A number of factors (outlined below) occurring simultaneously are considered critical in determining the likelihood of transmitting tubercle bacilli, of developing the infection, and of ultimately developing TB. Depending on the mix of factors in any given situation, the risk may be significant or insignificant (274).

Factors Influencing the Probability of Acquiring Tuberculous Infection

Most of the factors that determine the risk of acquiring tuberculous infection are environmental. By contrast, the risk of developing active TB after tuberculous infection is considered to be largely an individual characteristic, determined by immunologic status and other physiologic factors (described below). The main factors in determining whether the initial tuberculous infection is likely to occur are listed below:

- Probability of coming into contact with someone with infectious TB.
- Closeness or intimacy of that contact.
- Duration of contact.
- Number of viable bacilli present in the air.
- Susceptibility of the uninfected individual.

- Environmental conditions (e.g., volume of airspace, ventilation with outside air, relative humidity, presence of sunlight).

Crowding, particularly in living quarters, increases both the probability of coming into contact with an infectious individual if one is present and the closeness of that contact (66). Various types of institutional residences (e.g., nursing homes, hospitals, prisons, jails, and homeless shelters) can provide circumstances conducive to the transmission of TB. Health care workers (HCWs) are necessarily at increased risk of coming into contact with infectious patients. Performance of certain cough-inducing medical procedures, such as, bronchoscopy and administration of aerosolized pentamidine, on patients with infectious TB can increase HCWs' risk of exposure to airborne tubercle bacilli (52).

Infection occurs at the point in time when an infectious particle is inhaled. However, the likelihood of inhaling that particle is dependent on the concentration of such particles in the air and the length of time spent breathing that air; the greater the exposure, the greater the likelihood that infection will result. Frequent or prolonged exposure to an infectious source case (e.g., months) is usually necessary for transmission to occur (113). According to data derived in the mid-1980s, on average, less than 30 percent of household members become infected while living with an infectious source case, but the risk is highly variable (27,249). Under extraordinary circumstances (when the concentration of infectious particles in the air is much higher than usual), exposures as brief as 2 hours have reportedly led to infection (8).

In any given situation, the infectiousness of the source case determines whether any period of exposure could result in transmission. Individuals with untreated active pulmonary or laryngeal TB,[2] an advanced stage of disease, evidence of tubercle bacilli in sputum samples, and who cough frequently without covering the mouth are considered to be prime sources of infection (180).

Those not posing a risk of infection to others include individuals with tuberculous infection (rather than active disease), individuals with active TB who have been receiving adequate treatment long enough to render them noninfectious, and individuals with extrapulmonary TB without any lung or airway involvement. Adequate antimicrobial treatment can quickly reduce and eventually eliminate the infectiousness of individuals with drug-susceptible TB (160,253). Although the exact period of time required for this change varies from one patient to another and cannot be predicted precisely, research suggests it is about 6 months or longer (211). Patients with drug-resistant TB can, in some cases, be treated effectively, although the period of infectiousness may be prolonged until an adequate combination of appropriate drugs is determined. Those with MDR-TB for whom available drugs are ineffective may remain persistently infectious to others.

There is no evidence that untreated MDR-TB is more contagious than untreated drug-susceptible TB (291). However, because of delays in diagnosing resistance patterns and initiating adequate treatment, patients with MDR-TB are more likely to remain infectious for longer periods, thereby increasing their potential to infect others (see chapter 5). In several recent outbreaks of MDR-TB in hospitals, HCWs who were exposed to undiagnosed, persistently infectious patients with MDR-TB were more likely to have shown a tuberculin skin test conversion, indicating recent tuberculous infection, than HCWs without such exposure (350). There is also no evidence that HIV-infected patients with pulmo-

[2] Transmission of TB from patients with extrapulmonary TB (TB in tissue other than the lung) is unusual but has been reported, e.g., through manipulation of lesions or processing of lesions in the hospital or laboratory. Transmission of TB has been traced to patients with skin ulcers, abscesses, or other open lesions containing large numbers of tubercle bacilli that may be released into the air during medical procedures such as surgical draining or wound care (106,144,310).

nary TB are more or less infectious than non-HIV-infected patients with pulmonary TB (50).

Little is known about specific host factors that influence susceptibility to tuberculous infection. At present, there is no firm evidence that HIV-infected individuals are more likely to acquire tuberculous infection, although the frequency and rapidity with which HIV-infected individuals developed active TB in several recent outbreaks raises the possibility of heightened susceptibility in some populations with HIV (69,77). Individuals who are already infected with tubercle bacilli are generally considered to be partially resistant to further infection, but reinfection has been documented (207).

The concentration of infectious particles in the air also determines the likelihood of infection. Normal indoor air currents keep such particles (referred to as "droplet nuclei") airborne for long periods of time and disperse them throughout a room or a building (7,252). Until they dehydrate naturally, they remain infectious. These particles remain suspended until they are removed or diluted by ventilation or air filtration, or possibly inactivated by ultraviolet (UV) irradiation (see chapter 4). The use of these and other infection control measures can reduce the risk of transmission in the presence of infectious individuals (359).

Factors Influencing the Development of Active TB After Infection

The risk of developing active TB is highest shortly after tuberculous infection occurs and declines thereafter. Accordingly, the risk of disease is highest in the most recently infected individuals, who can be identified through contact investigation. The observed incidence of TB among those with positive tuberculin skin tests differs widely among populations studied, for reasons that are still unclear (66). Some evidence also indicates that the risk of infection is higher among those exposed to the most infectious cases and those with the closest contact to such cases (66).

Ninety percent of adults with tuberculous infection do not develop active TB, apparently due to the ability of their immune systems to hold the infection in check. Impairment of immune function (as in acquired immune deficiency syndrome (AIDS), by treatment with glucocorticoid or immunosuppressive drugs, malnutrition, various infections, or chronic conditions such as asthma and emphysema) tips the balance in favor of development of active TB among those with tuberculous infection (278,378). Whereas only 3 to 5 percent of immunocompetent individuals who acquire new tuberculous infection are thought to develop active TB within the first year after infection (97), the percent of HIV-infected individuals who acquire new infection and go on to develop active TB within the first year is estimated to be far greater (77). In a recent report, approximately one-third of the HIV-infected individuals sharing a residential facility who became infected with tubercle bacilli developed TB within 120 days (69). Most cases of TB among HIV-infected individuals are believed, however, to result from reactivation of latent tuberculous infection, rather than progression of recently acquired infection (278), although recent data from New York City indicates that the latter is increasing.

DEVELOPMENT OF TUBERCULOSIS AND ITS CLINICAL MANIFESTATIONS

Active TB manifests in a variety of ways, depending in part on the primary site of infection in the body. Pulmonary TB is the most common form of the disease, leading to cavity formation and progressive destruction of lung tissue. Pathologic and inflammatory processes associated with the disease produce weakness, fever, chest pain, cough, and when a small blood vessel is eroded, bloody sputum (31).

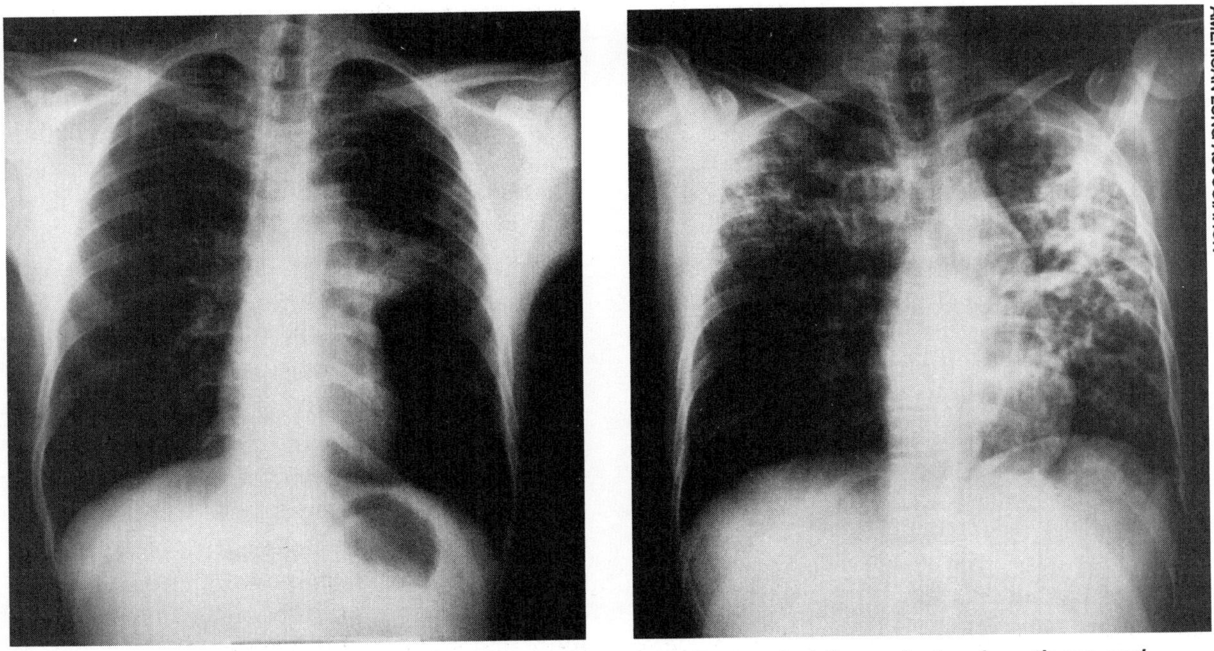

AMERICAN LUNG ASSOCIATION

TB, caused by an airborne bacillus, primarily affects the lungs. If untreated, it can destroy lung tissue and spread to other parts of the body and to the outside air. Pictured above are x-rays of a slightly diseased lung (left) and an extremely diseased lung (right).

The disease can affect other sites in the body (''extrapulmonary TB''), although only pulmonary and laryngeal TB are contagious through the airborne route. Various forms of extrapulmonary TB are more likely to occur in HIV-infected individuals and in children. These disseminated forms of the disease can result in the formation of small miliary (seed-like) lesions or life-threatening meningitis (inflammation of the membranes surrounding the brain and spinal cord). Such dissemination begins in the lung, which is the initial site of infection, and travels through the bloodstream to other parts of the body or through lymphatics to regional lymph nodes. Some organs take up and allow the multiplication of bacilli more readily than others, e.g., upper lung, kidneys, bone, and brain. Long-term damage can result, even in cured cases of TB, including impaired breathing due to lung damage, mental impairment from meningitis, and spinal deformity and leg weakness due to vertebral involvement (152).

Immune Responses to Tuberculous Infection and Disease

The cellular immune system is believed to play a central role in the development of TB in the body. While some of the relevant immunologic processes have been identified, fundamental questions remain concerning the interplay and regulation of immunologic forces that both inhibit the progress of the disease and actually contribute to the destructive disease process itself (31,74).

Airborne particles containing tubercle bacilli that are inhaled (and that manage to reach the lower parts of the lung) are initially engulfed by macrophages (a type of scavenger cell) in the alveoli (terminal air sacs in the lung). If the bacilli are not destroyed by the alvcolar macrophages, the bacilli multiply, killing the cell and attracting nonactivated macrophages from the bloodstream. In these new macrophages, the bacilli multiply logarithmically. Antigenic substances present within or secreted by tubercle bacilli stimulate T-lymphocytes (CD4 cells) to produce chemical substances (lymphokines), which activate these new macrophages, enabling them to destroy or inhibit the bacilli. The process by which macrophages are armed to destroy the bacilli they ingest is called cell-mediated immunity (CMI) and forms one part of the body's immune response to TB.

Another interrelated immune process that occurs in response to tuberculous infection is called delayed-type hypersensitivity (DTH), an inflammatory response that destroys bacilli-laden unactivated macrophages. An overabundance of DTH is blamed for most of tissue damage characteristic of pulmonary tuberculosis: caseous necrosis (death of tissues, leading to caseating granulomas and liquefaction of solid caseous tissue, producing cavities in the tissue) (71,72,73,74). Within the liquefied caseum, tubercle bacilli multiply outside of the cells, reaching tremendous numbers. Host resistance may be overwhelmed and the bacilli may develop resistance to antimicrobial drugs. Liquefaction and cavity formation allow the disease to become contagious, because the bacilli spread via the airways to other parts of the body and to the outside air.

Clinical Course in HIV-Seropositive Individuals

HIV-related immunodeficiency impairs both parts (DTH and CMI) of the immunologic response to tuberculous infection, leaving individuals with HIV more vulnerable to the development of clinical TB. Recent evidence suggests that TB tends to occur early in the course of HIV infection (321) often as the first overt manifestation of HIV infection. Infection with (non-contagious) non tuberculous mycobacteria, e.g., *Mycobacterium avium* complex, occurs frequently in individuals with AIDS, often leading to serious complications and earlier death. The surveillance definition of AIDS was recently expanded to include TB as an AIDS-defining condition among those with HIV infection (364).

The clinical course of TB in individuals with AIDS is dramatically different from TB in immunocompetent adults. Pulmonary TB in individuals with AIDS resembles that of TB in infants. The bacilli disseminate (via the bloodstream and lymphatics), producing extrapulmonary lesions, including tuberculous lymphadenitis or meningitis. Characteristic features of TB in individuals with HIV infection include a high prevalence of anergy to tuberculin skin testing (see chapter 4), atypical x-ray presentation of the disease in the lung, and frequency of extrapulmonary disease (162).

Clinical Course in Children

Infants and young children also manifest TB differently from immunocompetent adults, but the specific reasons for this are not yet clearly defined. Infants and young children can or are more likely to develop severe, life-threatening TB as an immediate complication of the primary infection, without the long latent period common in adults. They are more likely to develop extrapulmonary forms of the disease, especially lymphadenitis, osteotuberculosis, and meningitis (251,301). Active TB in such children typically is manifested by caseous lesions that do not liquefy or cavitate, so they are less likely to transmit the disease to others.

The Changing Epidemiology of Tuberculosis 3

After decades of steady decline in the number of new cases each year, tuberculosis (TB) is now on the increase in the United States. This turnabout has received considerable attention in the news media, medical literature, and public health sector. Reports of clusters of TB cases, particularly the more dangerous multidrug-resistant (MDR-TB) forms occurring recently in several hospitals and prisons, have been highlighted. These reports raise the specter of a serious, accelerating public health problem with the potential to spread regionally and nationally. For a disease that was widely considered to have been headed toward elimination in this country, the resurgence seems surprising and disturbing.

While many of the basic features of TB and its transmission are the same as those described decades ago, there are new elements that have changed the nature and magnitude of the problem. This chapter reviews current epidemiologic features of TB in the United States, including overall incidence, high-risk groups in the population, rates of coinfection with human immunodeficiency virus (HIV), and the cases of MDR-TB. Although the focus is on TB in the United States, some international data are included for comparison. Various factors that may be responsible for the recent changes in TB are discussed at the end of the chapter.

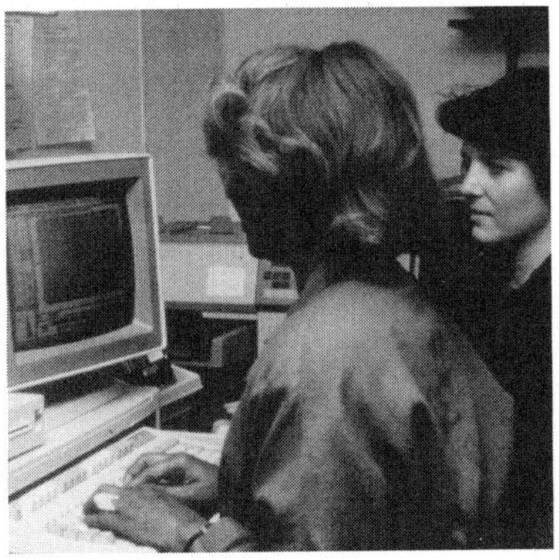

OVERALL TRENDS IN TB INCIDENCE

In 1953, the U.S. Public Health Service began a nationwide reporting system for TB, based on annual summaries of total TB cases reported in each State. In 1979, the Centers for Disease Control (CDC) began to phase in the "Report of a Verified Case of Tuberculosis" (RVCT) surveillance system, based on individ-

Figure 3-1—Reported Tuberculosis Cases in the United States, 1953-92

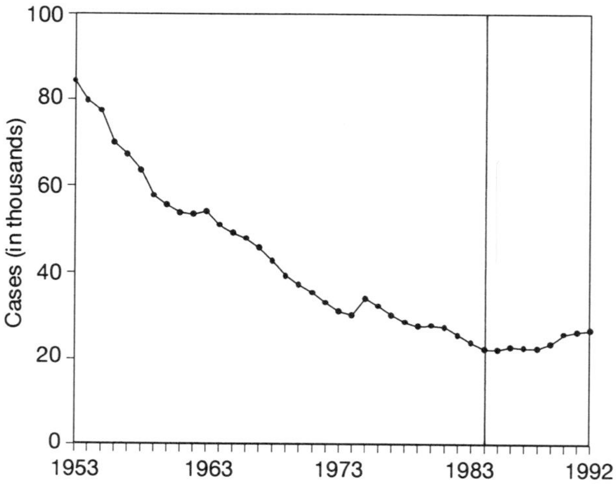

SOURCE: Office of Technology Assessment, 1993, based on data from U.S. Department of Health and Human Services, Public Health Service, Centers for Disease Control and Prevention, 1992.

ual case reports from all 50 States, the District of Columbia, and New York City (159).[1] The system was fully implemented in 1985. By using a standardized case definition and collecting data on individuals with TB (including age, sex, race, ethnicity, and country of origin), the RVCT system permitted a more detailed picture of TB epidemiology in the United States than was previously possible with aggregate data. In general, incidence rates based on case reports underestimate the true incidence of a disease, since many factors can influence the likelihood that any given case will actually be reported. It is unlikely that changing the TB reporting requirements in the RVCT system affected the overall ascertainment of cases, although it clearly produced more information about each case reported. The increased number of cases reported since the mid-1980s is much greater than could be accounted for by changes in the reporting system. In fact, significant underreporting of TB may still be occurring (28,250,307).

In 1953, there were 84,304 reported cases of TB, equivalent to a case rate of 53.0/100,000 population (27). Over the next 31 years, incidence declined steadily, with a few exceptions,[2] to 22,255 new cases in 1984 (case rate of 9.4/100,000 population) (233). The rate of decline averaged about 6 percent per year between 1953 and 1974, and about 5 percent per year between 1975 and 1984 (159,249). By 1984, the incidence of TB had declined 74 percent from its 1953 level (see figure 3-1).

This longstanding downward trend began to change in 1985. First, the decline in incidence slowed to just 0.2 percent in 1985, and then increased by 2.6 percent in 1986. Then, in 1987 and 1988 the decline in new cases resumed, but by only 1.1 and 0.4 percent, respectively. Further increases occurred in 1989 (4.7 percent), 1990 (the largest to date, 9.4 percent), 1991 (2.3 percent), and 1992 (1.5 percent) (334b). The number of reported cases in 1991 was 26,283 (case rate of 10.4/100,000), and in 1992 it was 26,673 (10.5/100,000) (353,356). This 1992 case total represented an 20 percent increase over 1985.

Averaged over the 6-year period, these data suggest a current upward trend of about 3 percent per year in cases, compared with the previous 5 to 6 percent annual decrease observed before 1984. Based on data indicating much sharper upturns in case rates in certain areas (see discussion below), it is possible that national rates may possibly continue to rise 2 percent per year, or go even higher, in the next decade.

DEMOGRAPHIC CHANGES IN TB

One of the most striking changes in TB epidemiology in the United States in recent decades has been a gradual shift in TB occurrence

[1] Data from Puerto Rico and the Virgin Islands are also collected, but are not referred to in the data cited in this report.

[2] A 1-year increase occurred in 1980 following a large influx of Indochinese refugees into the United States, and artificial increases were recorded in 1963 and 1975 due to changes in reporting criteria.

Figure 3-2—Rates of New Tuberculosis Cases in the United States, by State, 1991

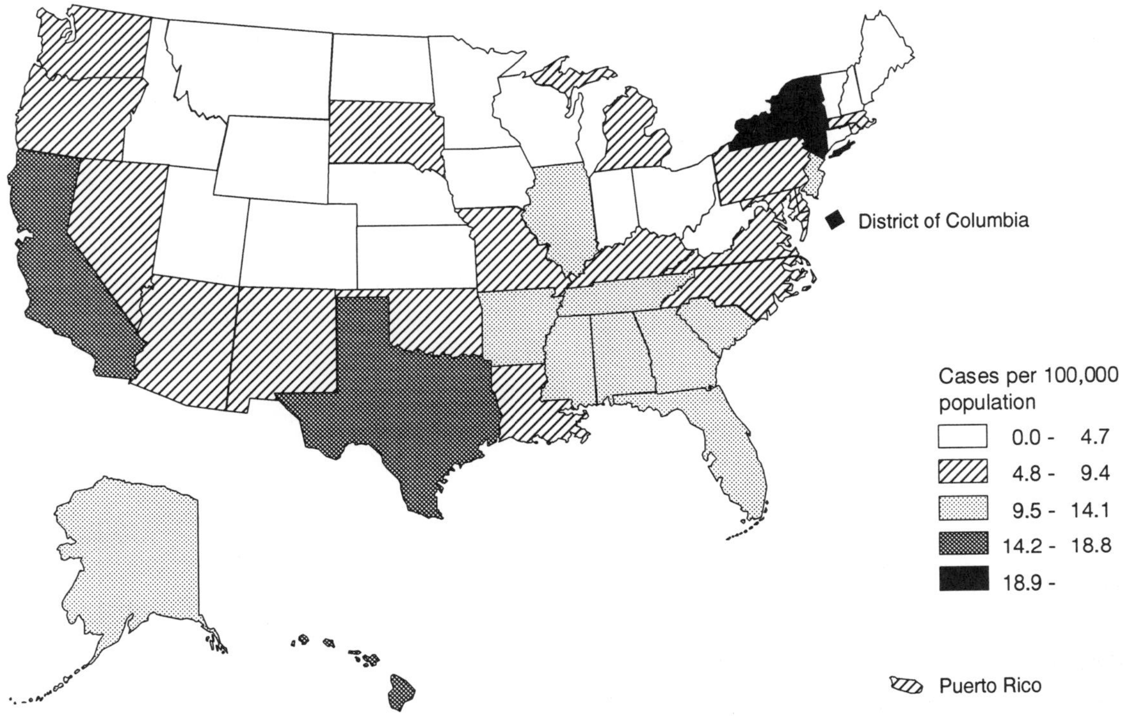

SOURCE: Office of Technology Assessment, 1993, based on data from U.S. Department of Health and Human Services, Public Health Service, Centers for Disease Control and Prevention, 1991.

from broader to narrower demographic populations (295), identified to some extent by geography, age, sex, race, ethnicity, and country of origin. A description of these changing characteristics can reveal where and in whom TB is occurring. It offers only limited information, however, about the epidemiology of the disease, since these characteristics are not causally related to TB; at best, they may be only indirectly associated with causal factors. Historically, TB has been linked primarily with environmental conditions that increase the likelihood of transmission, such as crowded, poorly ventilated housing and working conditions. Current data, described below, indicate that TB now occurs disproportionately among individuals who lack stable housing, abuse intravenous drugs or alcohol, become incarcerated, or are employed as migrant farm workers. A common element in these cases may also be environmental. The increasing occurrence of TB among individuals with HIV reflects a causal risk factor due to immunosuppression, as well as lifestyle factors such as drug abuse.

This section describes the current distribution of TB among demographic groups and summarizes the available data on the prevalence of TB in some high-risk populations. The epidemiologic association between TB and HIV is discussed later in the chapter.

Geographic Distribution

In 1991, more than half of the Nation's new cases came from five of the most populous States—California, New York, Texas, Florida, and Illinois (334). The highest TB case rates (the number of cases per 100,000 population), however, are found not only in these States but also in many smaller ones (see figure 3-2). New York

State ranked highest with a case rate of 24.5. Twelve other States recorded case rates above the national average of 10.4 for the same year: in descending order, Hawaii, California, Texas, Georgia, Florida, New Jersey, Alaska, Arkansas, Mississippi, Tennessee, South Carolina, and Alabama. The Southern region as a whole has long been above the national average in TB case rates (235). The lowest rates in 1991 were found in New Hampshire, Wyoming, North Dakota, Idaho, Nebraska, and Vermont (334).

Large urban areas as a group account for a disproportionate number of TB cases. In 1991, cities over 250,000 population accounted for 18 percent of the population, but more than 43 percent of new TB cases. About 14 percent of the Nation's cases came from New York City alone. The other major urban centers accounted for a much smaller percent of cases; Los Angeles, the city with the second highest number of new cases, accounted for about 4 percent of the Nation's cases, while Chicago, with the third highest, less than 3 percent (334a).

The ranking of cities by TB case rate indicates where TB is most concentrated. In 1991, the highest case rates were noted in Atlanta (76.4), Newark (71.8), New York City (50.3), Miami (48.5), and San Francisco (46.0) (see figure 3-3) (334a). Philadelphia and Chicago had relatively fewer cases, given their population size.

Some of the cities with currently high TB case rates have consistently had a high burden of TB for many years, even while the U.S. average case rates were declining. For example, figure 3-4

Figure 3-3—Highest and Lowest Rates of Active Tuberculosis in U.S. Cities of 250,000 or More, 1991

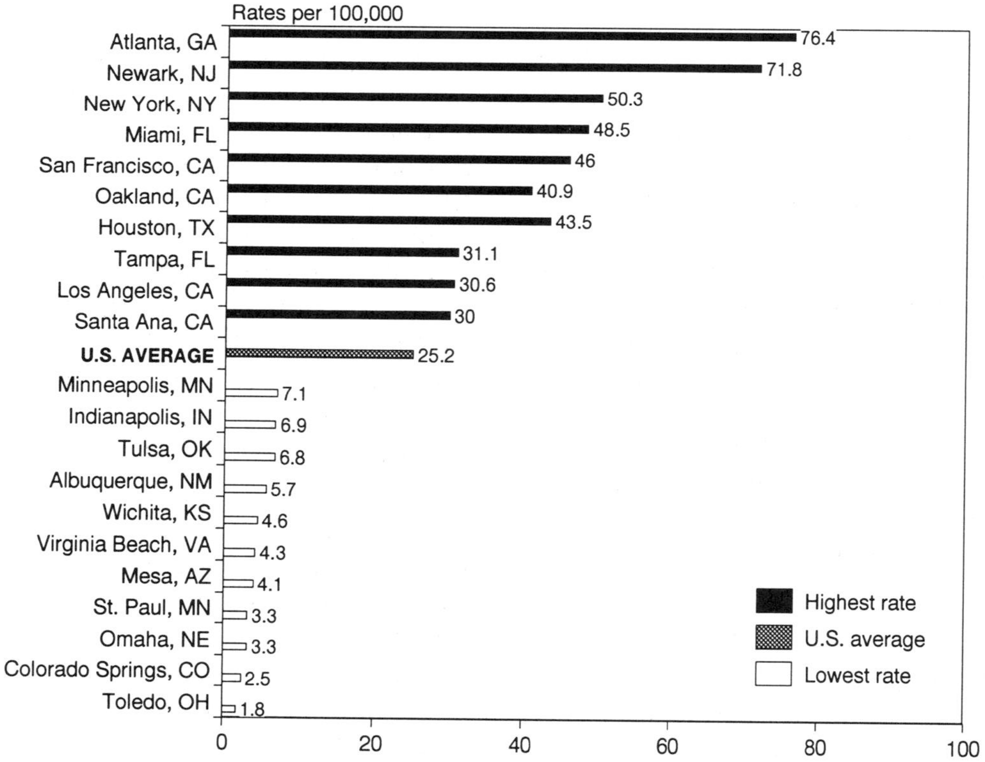

SOURCE: Office of Technology Assessment, 1993, based on data from U.S. Department of Health and Human Services, Public Health Service, Centers for Disease Control and Prevention, 1991.

Figure 3-4—U.S. Localities With Highest Tuberculosis Case Rates Compared With U.S. National Rates, 1969-91

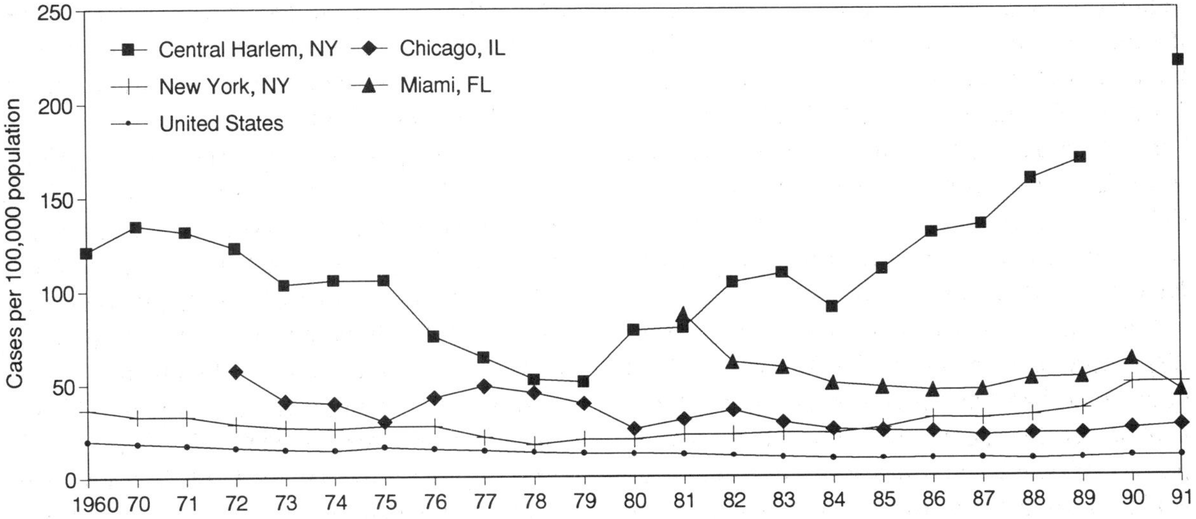

SOURCES: Office of Technology Assessment, 1993, based on data from Janice M. Burr, Medical Director of Tuberculosis Control Program, Dade County Department of Health, Miami, FL, personal communication, 1993; John Kuharik, Director, Tuberculosis Program, Chicago Department of Health, Chicago, IL, personal communication, 1993; K. Brudney and J. Dobkin, "Resurgent Tuberculosis in New York City: Human Immunodeficiency Virus, Homelessness, and the Decline of Tuberculosis Control Programs," *American Review of Respiratory Disease* 144:745-749, 1991.

shows TB case rates in Central Harlem New York City, (one of the areas of New York with the highest case rates), Chicago, and Miami, along with the national average rates since 1969 (45). Although the downward trend in U.S. rates began to change in the mid-1980s, case rates in New York City began to rise in 1979, and in Miami and Chicago, in the late 1980s; all three cities have been dealing with case rates well above the national average for many years. The exceptionally high rates of TB in Central Harlem all through the 1970s and 1980s show that TB remained endemic for decades even while the disease was receding nationally, presumably moving toward elimination (128).

Race, Ethnicity, Age, and Sex

Historically, TB in the United States has been most prevalent among ethnic and racial minorities living in impoverished areas (245), and today this trend still holds. In 1991, 71 percent of new cases occurred in racial and ethnic minorities (see figure 3-5). From 1985 to 1991, relatively large increases in numbers of TB cases occurred among Hispanic Americans (increasing 72 percent), Americans of Asian or Pacific Islands origin (increasing 32 percent), and black Americans (increasing 26 percent). During the same period, reports of cases decreased among non-Hispanic white Americans 9 percent and among Native Americans, 13 percent (293). Approximately two-thirds of cases in 1991 were reported in males, although the percent increase was slightly higher for females than males (293).

TB cases and rates generally increase with age, except among 5- to 14-year-olds, who have the lowest case rate of all age groups (159). Since 1985, however cases increased in all age groups except for those 65 or older. The largest increase by far, however, occurred among the 25- to 44-year-olds, who now constitute 39 percent of all cases (see figure 3-6) (293).

A comparison of the age distribution of cases divided according to race and ethnicity (see figure

Figure 3-5—Racial and Ethnic Distribution of Tuberculosis Cases in the United States, 1991

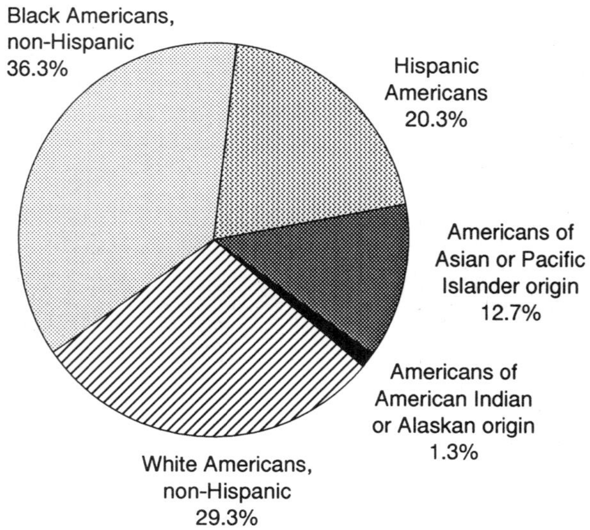

SOURCE: Office of Technology Assessment, 1993, based on data from U.S. Department of Health and Human Services, Public Health Service, Centers for Disease Control and Prevention, 1991.

3-7) shows a dramatically different pattern among whites compared to black Americans and Hispanic Americans. Among white Americans, the majority of cases occur among elderly individuals, while among black and Hispanic Americans, an increasing number of cases is occurring among young adults in the 25- to 44-age-group. Minorities are disproportionately represented, particularly in this age group; of the 10,263 cases reported in 1991 among 25- to 44-year-olds, 45 percent occurred among black Americans, 22 percent among Hispanic Americans, 19 percent among white Americans, and 13 percent among Americans of Asian or Pacific Islands origin (293).

Children

Unlike cases among adults, TB among children is evidence of recent transmission of the disease—suggesting the presence of other individuals (usually adults) with active, infectious TB in the community (163,302,307). While transmission to children could occur in group settings such as family homes, schools, family day care homes, or nursery schools, a large TB clinic in Houston traced 80 percent of the cases to an infectious adult contact in the child's household (302). In some areas of the country, immigration from countries with high rates of TB may also account for high rates of TB among children.

Nationally, new cases of TB in children declined an average of 6 percent annually from 1962 until 1987, but then began to rise in 1988. In 1991, 1,662 new cases were reported in children under 15 years of age, an increase of 32 percent over 1985; most of the increase occurred among Hispanic American children, so that in 1991 Hispanic Americans accounted for nearly half of all cases in children. Overall, 86 percent of cases occurred in racial and ethnic minorities, compared with 80 percent in 1985 (302). Cases declined, however, not only among white American children, but also among Americans of Asian or Pacific Islands origin, American Indian, and Alaskan Native children during this period (293).

Figure 3-6—Reported Tuberculosis Cases in the United States by Age, 1985 and 1991

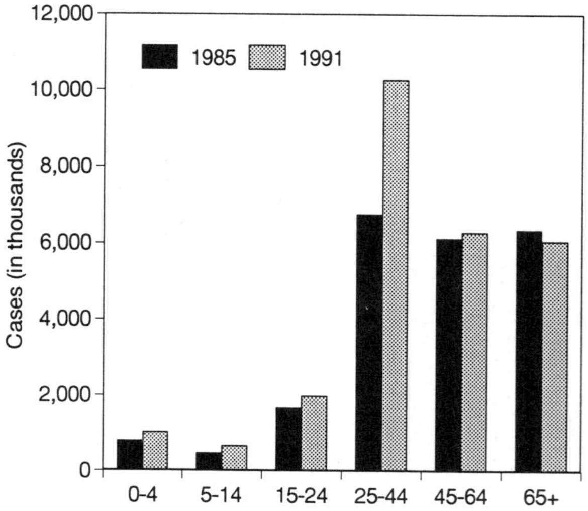

SOURCE: Office of Technology Assessment, 1993, based on data from U.S. Department of Health and Human Services, Public Health Service, Centers for Disease Control and Prevention, 1991.

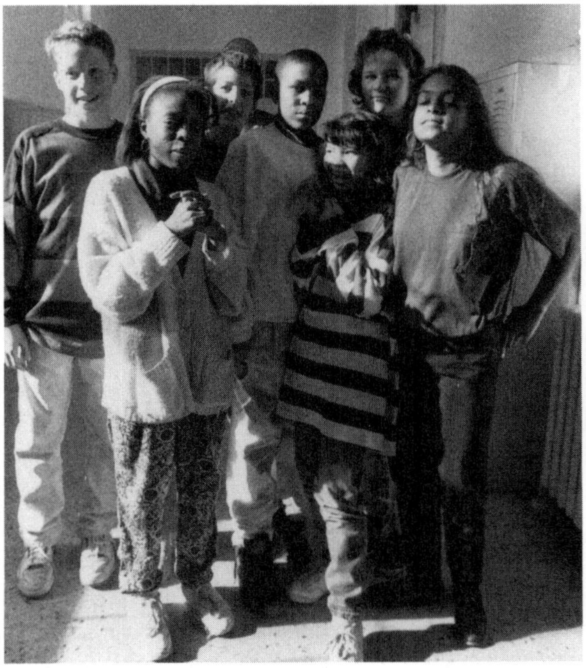

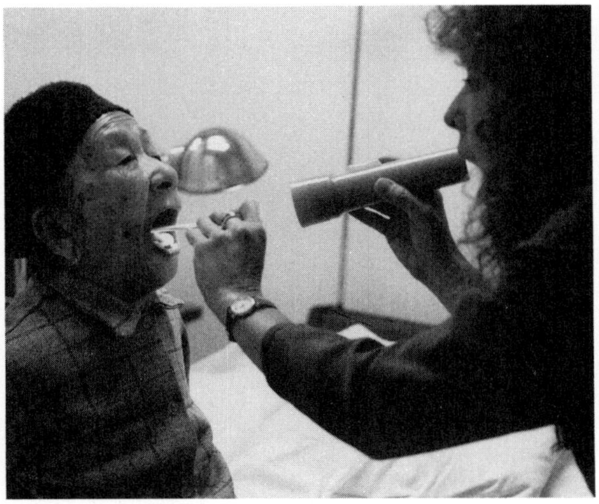

BENJAMIN SMITH and ON LOK SENIOR HEALTH SERVICES

Individuals at high risk of TB in the United States include elderly people and economically-disadvantaged people, especially those who are members of racial and ethnic minority groups, children, and those born in other countries.

Figure 3-7—U.S. Tuberculosis Cases Among Black and Hispanic Americans Compared With Non-Hispanic White Americans, 1985, 1987, 1989 and 1990

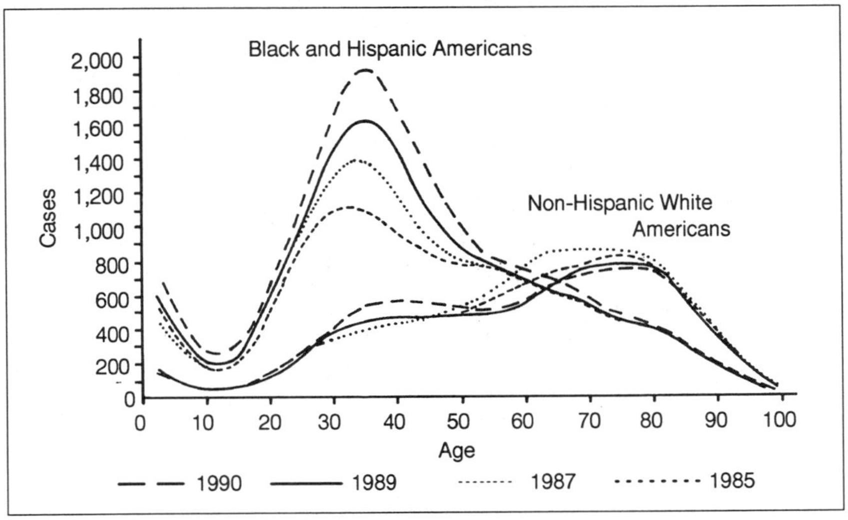

SOURCE: M.E. Villarino, L.J. Geiter, and P.M. Simone, "The Multidrug-Resistant Tuberculosis Challenge to Public Health Efforts to Control Tuberculosis," *Public Health Reports* 107(6):616-625, 1992.

In 1991, three States contributed almost 60 percent of the cases among children: California (with 563 cases), Texas (with 219 cases), and New York (with 198 cases). Large percent increases in recent years, however, occurred in New Jersey and Arizona (293). High rates of TB among immigrants such as in California and increases in TB among parents of the 25 to 44 age group may account for the observed increases among children.

Elderly Individuals

In 1991, elderly individuals accounted for nearly a quarter of all new TB cases; the case rate among individuals 65 or older is currently the highest of any age group (358). The vast majority of these cases result from infection acquired earlier in life when TB was more prevalent, with the infection then progressing to active disease in older age (311). Some evidence suggests, however, that some TB cases among the elderly individuals result from recent infection or active transmission (309,311). Residents of nursing homes or other long-term care facilities may be at greater risk for TB than those living in single family homes (312). Data from a CDC survey of over 15,000 TB cases among elderly individuals living in nursing homes compared with noncongregate sites between 1984 and 1985 showed an annual case rate in nursing homes nearly twice as high (358). A smaller, more intensive survey among cases reported in Arkansas suggested an even higher relative risk for nursing home residents (312).

High-Risk Populations

Immigrants and Refugees

As a group, U.S. residents born outside of the United States tend to have higher rates of TB than those born in this country (360). This trend reflects the fact that TB is more prevalent in many areas of the world, particularly regions of Asia, Africa, and Latin America, than in the United States (199,316). In 1991, 27 percent of the 6,982 new cases were reported among the foreign-born; this is increased from 22 percent in 1986 (293).

The vast majority of these cases were reported in people of either Hispanic, Asian, or Pacific Islands origin. Such cases made up sizable proportions of all cases within each of these ethnic groups: 55 percent of all Hispanic American cases and 89 percent of all cases among Americans of Asian or Pacific Island origin were reported as foreign-born in 1991 (293).

Residents of Homeless Shelters

Various surveys among selected clinics and shelters serving homeless individuals indicate that the prevalence of active TB may range from 2 to 7 percent (184,275,289). The prevalence is likely to be highly variable, however, depending on the site, population, and time period studied. The proportion of TB patients who are also homeless may be high. In New York City, 20 percent of new TB cases reported in 1991 were also identified as homeless, based on a computerized matching of shelter addresses to TB cases in the registry (57).

There are several factors that make homeless individuals generally more vulnerable to development of active TB. The prevalence of tuberculous infection among homeless individuals is reported to be quite high—up to 50 percent in some studies (16,184,285,289,342). Factors predisposing homeless individuals with TB infection to progress to active disease include impaired immunity (due to poor nutrition, poor health status overall, substance abuse, and/or HIV infection) and lack of access to preventive treatment (184).

In addition, homeless shelters typically provide ideal conditions for transmission of tuberculous infection—large numbers of people in close proximity, poor ventilation, the presence of undiagnosed or untreated infectious cases, and prolonged exposure due to lengthy stays particularly in winter months (325). Studies have also shown that previously infected residents may also become reinfected in the shelter and progress rapidly to active disease (207). In recent years, several outbreaks of TB disease in homeless shelters have been reported (207,212,342,351).

Drug Users

Drug users are another population that overlaps with several other identifiable groups at high risk for TB, particularly the HIV-infected and homeless. Results of a recent study of MDR-TB in New York City indicated that intravenous drug use was an independent risk factor for the development of MDR-TB in that population (107). A survey conducted in the early 1970s of drug-dependent individuals identified through New York City drug addiction treatment centers and methadone maintenance treatment programs showed a high prevalence of TB in this population (246). A recent report documented an outbreak of TB among crack cocaine users in Contra Costa County, California (349). In 283 cases of TB reported during a 42-month period, 16 percent (44 individuals) were found to have occurred among crack cocaine users. Fifteen of the 44 drug users frequented one or more crack houses, environments that may facilitate active transmission of TB. Crack use, which damages the lungs and promotes coughing, can lead to increased active transmission of TB among users in close quarters and in poorly ventilated surroundings typical of crack houses. No direct link of crack use in the risk of infection was documented.

Prisoners and Inmates

The prevalence of TB in correctional institutions (including prisons, jails, and detention centers) is related both to the prevalence of tuberculous infection and HIV in the incarcerated population and to conditions within the institutions favoring spread of tuberculous infection. On both accounts, TB has become a significant and increasing health problem within the correctional system (23). These factors are an issue not only for the correctional system itself (with its average daily population of 1.2 million in 1990) (112), but for the country as a whole, since inmates who develop TB within the system carry it with them into the community following release (308); in addition, correctional staff who become infected and develop active TB can, in turn, transmit the disease to their family and other contacts in the community (346).

Population groups at high risk for TB—individuals who abuse drugs, who are HIV-infected, and who are homeless—are disproportionately represented in the correctional system (112,346). In the New York State system, 26 percent of the women and 16 percent of the men were also found to be HIV-infected in a recent blinded serosurvey. Almost one-third of newly admitted inmates in New York State reported having been homeless just prior to incarceration, and the majority of inmates had histories of substance abuse (209).

TB may be at least three times more prevalent among inmates and prisoners than in nonincarcerated adults (335). In the New York State, New Jersey, and California correctional systems, for example, the prevalence of TB in the mid-1980s was 6 to 11 times higher than in the general population of those States (41,346). In New York State, the incidence of TB began rising in the early 1980s (before any coinfections with HIV were identified) but accelerated its rise in 1986; it increased four-fold from under 25 cases per 100,000 in the late 1970s to over 100 per 100,000 in 1986. Approximately one-half of the cases between 1985 and 1986 were found to have HIV infection, based on a study matching TB and AIDS registries. Most TB cases were in minority men between 30- and 49-years-old with histories of intravenous drug use (41).

Since 1985, at least 11 outbreaks of TB have occurred in correctional institutions in eight States (346); the most recent one involved a cluster of MDR-TB cases in which 13 inmates and one correctional officer died of the disease. The presence of inmates with active, infectious disease in close proximity with large numbers of highly susceptible individuals in poorly ventilated surroundings creates a scenario for rapid and widespread infection (308). Frequent transfers of prisoners within and between facilities may also serve to broaden the scope of the problem.

Migrant Farm Workers

Evidence suggests that migrant farm workers,[3] many of whom are immigrants from counties with a high prevalence of TB, may also be at high risk

[3] Migrant farm workers are defined as seasonal agricultural workers who move from area to area for jobs.

for TB. A 1988 study of 543 migrant farm workers in North Carolina found an overall prevalence of active TB in 2 percent of workers (0.47 percent in Hispanic American workers and 3.6 percent in black American workers), along with high rates of TB infection (33 percent of Hispanic Americans, 54 percent of black Americans, and 76 percent of Haitian immigrants) (55). High rates of tuberculous infection have also been noted in other migrant worker populations (296,362). Since there is no regular monitoring of this population, the overall prevalence of TB in the U.S. migrant farm worker population is unknown.

Data from the North Carolina study suggest that TB in migrant farm workers may be at least partly an occupational problem, since those with longer migrant work histories had greater risks of TB. Lack of access to health services and substandard working and housing conditions are likely factors in this heightened risk. Characteristics of the migrant population also predispose them to TB. A high percentage of workers, mostly black Americans, are recruited from homeless shelters, soup kitchens, and alcohol rehabilitation centers. While immigrants (generally from Central America, Mexico, and Haiti) constitute a large part of the migrant work force, the North Carolina study found much higher rates of TB disease among U.S.-born black workers compared with the foreign-born workers (55).

HIV AND AIDS: EPIDEMIOLOGIC ASSOCIATION WITH TB

Reports in the mid-1980s were the first to describe an association between TB and AIDS, based on clinical studies of Haitian immigrants in Florida (231) and intravenous drug users (IVDUs) in New Jersey (319). In recent years, a significant physiologic interaction between the two infections has become clear. This interaction is relevant not only to the medical care of individuals coinfected with tubercle bacilli and HIV, but also to the resurgence of TB in many areas.

Current evidence indicates that HIV-related immunosuppression impairs the body's ability to contain infection with tuberculous mycobacteria. As a result, individuals infected with TB and HIV, particularly those with advanced immunosuppression, are at high risk of progressing rapidly to active TB disease; this is true whether they have recently become infected with TB or previously harbored the latent TB infection (69,77,81,278). Rapid progression to active TB disease among individuals with AIDS seems to be a more dangerous course of TB, with death often occurring before treatment for TB begins or within the first month of treatment (290). The estimated annual risk of progression to active TB disease among dually-infected individuals has been estimated to be as high as 8 percent per year (278), compared with an average risk among HIV-seronegative individuals of 10 percent per lifetime.

In addition, preliminary observations suggest some individuals with HIV infection may be more likely than a healthy individual to acquire the initial TB infection after contact with someone who has active, infectious TB (69). Heightened susceptibility and prolonged periods of infectivity have been cited as potential factors in several recent outbreaks of MDR-TB among HIV-infected individuals in congregate settings (48,69,77,81,195).

An estimated 10 million people in the United States are infected with tubercle bacilli (248) and an estimated 1 million are infected with HIV. As has been seen in some areas, the presence of HIV can profoundly affect the incidence of TB, particularly where populations with TB and HIV overlap to a large extent (202,229,249,315). According to a recent CDC analysis of trends in reported cases of TB among U.S.-born individuals between 1985 and 1991, the largest increases in numbers of TB cases were found in groups of States with the highest incidence of AIDS (defined as 138 to 636/100,000 population); TB incidence was found to have declined in States with the lowest cumulative AIDS incidence (5 to

46/100,000), and remained at the same level in those with an intermediate incidence of AIDS (48 to 97/100,000) (293). These data suggest that HIV may be having a direct impact on TB, accounting for at least some of the resurgence of TB in these areas. Common factors, such as the occurrence of both diseases in some of the same demographic groups, may also be contributing to the observed association. Inmates and IVDUs, for example, are at higher risk for TB than the general population because a greater proportion of individuals in these groups have tuberculous infection and are also at high risk for HIV infection; in addition, noninfected inmates and IVDUs are also at high risk for TB due to the potential for transmission within correctional facilities, crack houses, and other settings (23,355).

A recent analysis of U.S. death certificates filed between 1980 and 1990 indicated an increase in deaths due to TB in young adults, believed to be associated with the AIDS epidemic. In 1990, more than half of the deaths with TB in individuals 20- to 49-years-old occurred in those who also had AIDS listed on their death certificates (39).

In developing countries, particularly in sub-Saharan Africa and Haiti where both AIDS and TB are more prevalent than in the United States, AIDS appears to be having a substantial impact on TB. According to World Health Organization (WHO) estimates, 4 million people worldwide are dually infected with tubercle bacilli and HIV, the majority of whom live in developing countries; as many as two-thirds of TB patients in some countries may be HIV-seropositive (236). Internationally, TB is one of the most common opportunistic infections of AIDS and is the AIDS-defining condition in about 30 percent of cases (132). This could lead to a dramatic increase in the number of deaths from TB over the next decade in regions where TB and AIDS are endemic (135,201).

The Prevalence of TB Among Individuals With AIDS

Studies of individuals with AIDS in the United States have consistently shown a higher prevalence of TB compared with the general population, even after adjustment for age, race, and sex (67,232). Overall, 4.9 percent of AIDS cases reported up to 1990 also appeared on TB registries, according to a CDC analysis of TB and AIDS registries in 43 States and 11 localities (293,344). Substantially higher prevalence rates of TB among individuals with AIDS have recently been reported in certain populations: for example, 26 percent of men with HIV infection and 40 percent of men with AIDS or AIDS-related complex living in a homeless shelter in New York City and 13 percent of patients with AIDS in a New York City hospital were found to have active TB (177,325). The 1990 overall proportion of 4.9 percent increased from 4.0 percent 2 years earlier (344).

Another indicator that the prevalence of TB may be increasing among individuals with AIDS is the disproportionate increase in the incidence of extrapulmonary TB, which rose by 20 percent nationwide, compared with pulmonary TB, which rose by 3 percent, between 1984 and 1989. Extrapulmonary TB is more often seen among individuals with AIDS (see chapter 2) (27,218).[4] *M.tb.* isolates may represent only 10 percent of mycobacterial infections in patients with AIDS, however. Infection with nontuberculous mycobacteria such as *M.avium* is very common among AIDS patients; these infections occur in later stages of AIDS (when CD4 cell counts are below 100/mm^3), are untreatable, and may be life-threatening.

[4] According to CDC's 1987 definition of AIDS, an HIV-infected individual with extrapulmonary TB would be reportable as AIDS (40). In 1993, this definition was broadened to include, among other conditions, pulmonary TB as a defining condition of AIDS among HIV-infected individuals with CD4+ lymphocyte counts under 200 cells/mm^3 (365).

MULTIDRUG-RESISTANT TUBERCULOSIS

Drug-resistant TB is not a new phenomenon, but in recent years, the predominant types of MDR-TB have changed, as has the overall number of cases in the United States.

Three general categories of drug resistance apply to TB, although, in practice, it is not always possible to determine which one applies in any given case: primary resistance, which is a naturally occurring biological phenomenon that rarely results in resistance to more than one drug, but also refers to a drug resistance in a patient not known to have received prior treatment; acquired resistance, which is a manmade problem caused by inadequate or erratic treatment and can result in resistance to one or more drugs in each case; and transmitted resistance, which occurs in active transmission to contacts from infectious cases (e.g., in institutional settings) and results in resistance to the same number and types of drugs as in the source case (154).[5]

Until the past several years, TB experts generally assumed that most cases of MDR-TB were acquired through inadequate or erratic treatment in an individual case. Increasingly, however, transmitted resistance is being implicated in reported cases of MDR-TB (48). For example, in New York City, a survey of all TB cases reported during April 1991 suggested that most patients with drug-resistant isolates had drug resistance because they were initially infected with resistant bacilli (107). Although both categories of resistance appear to be important at present, the actual proportion of each in the U.S. population is unknown. Genetic fingerprinting technology has recently been used to track the spread of specific strains of tubercle bacilli among infected individuals in an outbreak situation, thus providing strong evidence of active transmission in certain cases (69).

From a public health standpoint, the most significant forms of drug-resistant TB are resistant to both isoniazid (INH) and rifampin (RIF), two of the most powerful anti-TB drugs. Such cases of MDR-TB are generally far more difficult and costly to treat than drug-sensitive TB, and can be fatal despite the best available treatment (see chapter 5 for further details).

The proportion of cases with drug-resistant TB in the United States, Canada, and Europe has traditionally been lower than in many other countries. In many areas of Latin America, Asia, and Africa, higher rates of TB overall, inadequate TB control programs, uncontrolled dispensing of drugs, and ineffective treatment delivery systems all contribute to higher rates of drug-resistant TB (156). On entry to the United States, immigrants from these areas can harbor tuberculous infection that may be drug-resistant.

Current national data on the incidence and prevalence of drug-resistant TB in the United States are unavailable because, until 1993, the TB surveillance system did not collect information on drug-susceptibility of reported cases (382). Although some States or communities regularly preform susceptibility testing on TB cases, others test only on some individuals on an optional basis (156). As of 1993, reports of each case of TB will be required to include drug susceptibility data (26). Since 1961, CDC conducted periodic national surveys of primary drug resistance, but discontinued the practice in 1986, partly due to evidence of stable or declining proportions of patients with drug resistance but also due to competing priorities for CDC resources. Several large national surveys conducted over the past few decades do offer some information on the epidemiology of drug-resistant TB in the United States.

---

[5] Although these definitions are accepted by most TB experts, the CDC uses a different scheme to distinguish among types of resistance. The CDC classification uses the term "primary resistance" to refer to all TB not previously treated; this category combines "primary" and "transmitted" resistance as they are defined in the text. The CDC's term "secondary resistance" is equivalent to "acquired resistance" as defined in the text.

Figure 3-8—Culture-Positive Cases of Tuberculosis Resistant to One or More Drugs, by Region, 1991

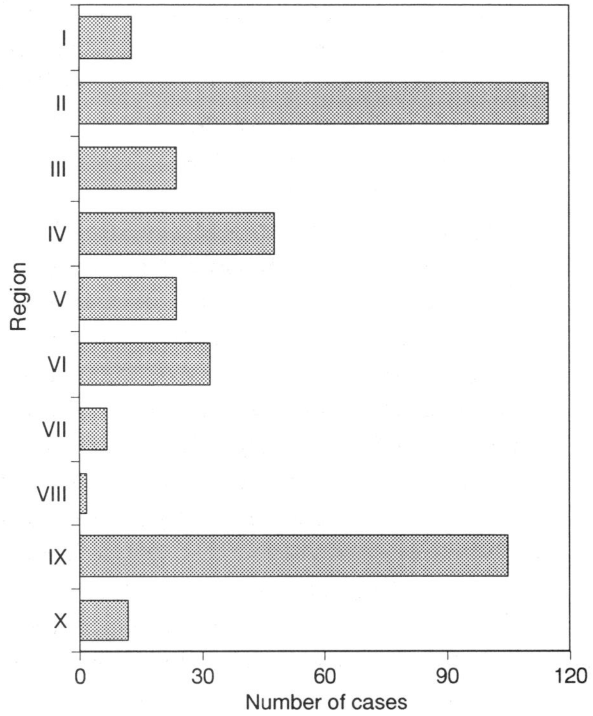

REGION I
Connecticut
Maine
Massachusetts
New Hampshire
Rhode Island

REGION II
New Jersey
New York
Puerto Rico
Virgin Islands

REGION III
Delaware
District of Columbia
Maryland
Pennsylvania
Virginia
West Virginia

REGION IV
Alabama
Florida
Georgia
Kentucky
Mississippi
North Carolina
South Carolina
Tennessee

REGION V
Illinois
Michigan
Minnesota
Ohio
Wisconsin

REGION VI
Arkansas
Louisiana
New Mexico
Oklahoma
Texas

REGION VII
Indiana
Kansas
Missouri
New England

REGION VIII
Colorado
Montana
North Dakota
South Dakota
Utah
Wyoming

REGION IX
Arizona
California
Hawaii
Nevada

REGION X
Alaska
Idaho
Oregon
Washington

SOURCE: Office of Technology Assessment, 1993, based on data from U.S. Department of Health and Human Services, Public Health Service, Centers for Disease Control and Prevention, 1991.

The incidence of primary resistance to anti-TB drugs remained under 3 percent from the 1940s, when antibiotics were first used to treat TB, through the 1960s (82). An average rate of primary resistance of 7.1 (range of 3.3 to 15.1 percent) was found in a national survey of over 7,500 patients tested in 19 city and State laboratories by CDC between 1975 and 1977, with higher rates found among Asian and Hispanic American patients than other racial and ethnic groups. Another survey of 20 State and city labs involving over 11,000 patients, conducted between 1975 and 1982, found a declining incidence of primary resistance over the period of the study, with a 6.9 percent rate overall and variation by geography, race, and ethnicity (172,338,340).

A higher average incidence of primary resistance to one or more drugs (9.0 percent) (with 0.5 percent resistant to two or more drugs during this same period) was found in a 1982-86 survey conducted by CDC, (based on 3,760 samples from 31 health departments across the country (51,297). Results showed a decreased rate of primary resistance during the 4-year survey. Because of different methods of sampling and data collection, however, results of the 1975-82 survey and the 1982-86 survey are not comparable.

More recent and comprehensive data are available from a nationwide CDC survey of drug resistance among new TB cases reported during the first 3 months of 1991. This survey did not include data on drug resistance in prevalent cases, so it provides only a minimal estimate on the number of drug-resistant cases in the United States. Provisional analysis of these data show that drug resistant TB is present in many areas of the country (see figure 3-8); cases resistant to at least one drug were reported from 36 States and to both INH and RIF from 13 States.

A total of 114 cases of TB in newly diagnosed cases resistant to both INH and RIF were found, with more than half of these reported from New York City.[6] Resistance to both INH and RIF was 3.5 percent, representing cases in which the two best anti-TB drugs could not be given. Overall, 14.2 percent of the cases had resistance to at least one drug (the majority to INH) (19,363).

Rates of drug-resistance among selected populations of TB patients have also been described (54). A recent study of drug resistance among TB cases reported in New York City gives an indication of the magnitude of the problem in that area. In a collaborative study with CDC, the New York City Department of Health conducted a systematic survey of TB cases to measure drug resistance among all patients in New York City who had a positive culture for TB during the month of April 1991 (107). Overall, 33 percent of cases were resistant to one or more drugs, and 19 percent were resistant to both INH and RIF.

Divided according to primary and acquired resistance, the study found that among cases not previously treated, 23 percent were resistant to one or more drugs and 7 percent to both INH and RIF; among those currently or previously treated, 44 percent were resistant to one or more drugs and 30 percent to both INH and RIF. The New York City Department of Health reported that for the entire year of 1991, a total of 366 new cases of TB resistant to both INH and RIF were reported in New York City—about 10 percent of all cases that year (57). No other area of the country currently has as high a level of MDR-TB. Further, limited evidence suggests that the prevalence of MDR-TB in New York is increasing. During a recent 3-year period at a large hospital center in Brooklyn, the prevalence of TB cases resistant to two or more drugs increased from 12 percent (31 cases per 265 patients) to 18 percent (39 cases per 221 patients) (280).

Recent Outbreaks of MDR-TB in Institutional Settings

Although community outbreaks of drug-resistant TB (237,339) are not an entirely new occurrence, a recent series of reports indicate that such outbreaks have become more common, larger in scope, and more dangerous.

Since 1990, CDC has investigated nine outbreaks of MDR-TB in the United States (370). At least seven additional clusters of drug-resistant TB, however, have been reported in 1990 and 1991 but not investigated by CDC (in Illinois, Mississippi, New York, and Michigan). They have occurred in several hospitals in New York City and Miami; in New York State and New Jersey; and in prison facilities in New York State (see table 3-1). The total number of individuals who developed active MDR-TB in these outbreaks had risen to 297 as of October 1992 (78). Most, though not all, were HIV-seropositive. The majority (79 to 89 percent) of the individuals affected by these outbreaks have died from the disease, including six health care workers and one prison guard; the median interval between diagnosis and death was just 4 to 16 weeks (363). Almost all cases were resistant to at least INH and RIF, and some to as many as seven drugs (80). It is not known whether the high rate of mortality observed in these outbreaks applies to other individuals with MDR-TB, whether or not they are HIV-infected.

In these institutional settings, MDR-TB was transmitted from patient to patient, from patient to health care worker, from inmate to inmate, and from inmate to prison staff. A number of common factors have been investigated as possible causes of the rapid transmission of the disease in these different settings (80). The immediate factor in

[6] Cases of TB resistant to both INH and RIF: 51 from New York City, 9 from New Jersey, 7 from Florida, 6 from California, 5 from Texas, 3 from Alabama, 3 from Illinois, and 1 each from Hawaii, Arizona, Virginia, Washington, Georgia, and Pennsylvania (26).

Table 3-1—Nosocomial HIV-Related Multidrug-Resistant Tuberculosis Outbreaks, 1988 to October 1992

Facility	Location	Time period	Total cases	Resistance pattern[a]
Hospital A	Miami	1988-91	65	INH, RIF (EMB, ETA)
Hospital B	New York City	1989-91	51	INH, SM (RIF, EMB)
Hospital C	New York City	1989-92	70	INH, RIF, SM (EMB, ETA, KM, RBT)
Hospital D	New York City	1990-91	29	INH, RIF (EMB, ETA)
Hospital E	New York State	1991	7	INH, RIF, SM (EMB, ETA, KM, RBT)
Hospital F	New York City	1990-91	16	INH, RIF, SM (EMB, ETA, KM, RBT)
Hospital I	New Jersey	1990-92	13	INH, RIF (EMB)
Hospital J	New York City	1991-92	28	INH, RIF (SM, EMB, ETA, KM)
Prison system[b]	New York State	1990-92	42	INH, RIF (SM, EMB, ETA, KM, RBT)
Total cases[b]			297	

KEY: EMB = Ethambutol; ETA = Ethionamide; HIV = human immunodeficiency virus; INH = Isoniazid; KM = Kanamycin; RBT = Rifabutin; RIF = Rifampin; SM = Streptomycin.

[a] All cases are resistant to first group of drugs listed. Some cases are also resistant to the drugs listed within the parentheses.

[b] 24 prison cases are also counted with Hospital C.

SOURCE: Office of Technology Assessment, 1993, based on data from U.S. Department of Health and Human Services, Public Health Service, Centers for Disease Control, 1992.

each case is the presence of individuals with active, infectious TB in close proximity to others; such patients remain infectious until at least several weeks into appropriate therapy under the best of circumstances, or, in untreatable cases, remain infectious indefinitely. Furthermore, delayed diagnosis and delayed initiation of appropriate therapy in treatable cases increase the chances of spreading the disease. For a number of reasons, HIV-seropositive individuals with MDR-TB may be more difficult to diagnose. In addition, drug susceptibility testing, which is necessary to assure an appropriate treatment regimen, usually takes several weeks to months to complete. Heightened vulnerability to the rapid development of active TB among HIV-seropositive individuals infected with tubercle bacilli also contribute to these outbreaks.

Delayed implementation of infection control measures, premature discontinuation of isolation, delayed reporting of drug-resistance, and lack of isolation facilities were major factors in the spread of MDR-TB within these institutions. Given the medical limitations cited above, infection control practices adequate to the task may be essential to prevent further spread of the disease in these circumstances (see chapter 5 for further details). In at least one setting where an outbreak occurred, the adoption of improved infection control practices was believed to be largely responsible for the absence of further cases of transmitted MDR-TB (20).

FACTORS UNDERLYING THE TB RESURGENCE IN THE UNITED STATES

Recent changes in the nature and magnitude of TB involve a broad range of interrelated factors. No one factor appears to be the predominant cause of the resurgence. Medical factors (such as HIV-related immunosuppression), social factors (e.g., homelessness and incarceration), and health policy issues (such as reduced resources for TB control in general) (see chapter 7) have all contributed to the problem in various ways (31).

One of the most basic and often overlooked reasons for the resurgence is inadequate control of the disease in some areas, even though its overall incidence steadily declined in the general population (277). The maintenance of a reservoir of TB permitted the larger resurgence to occur when conditions favored its spread. Certain communities in New York City, such as Central Harlem, are examples of areas where TB rates remained consistently high in the 1960s and 1970s compared with regional and national rates. The incidence of TB in Harlem began to rise in the late 1970s (before AIDS became prevalent and well before national TB rates began to rise). The rise was driven by a variety of factors, particularly homelessness, intravenous drug use, and the decline of TB control programs (45). TB rates began to increase more quickly in Harlem in the mid-1980s, as HIV became prevalent in the same population (57).

Social and public policy issues figure prominently in the resurgence. Some of the most intractable social problems are generally believed to play a role, directly or indirectly, in furthering the spread of TB, including, poverty, homelessness, substance abuse, poor health status, language barriers, and crowded, substandard living conditions. The AIDS epidemic in some of the same populations provided the vehicle for an accelerated rate of increase in TB. Immigration of individuals from certain countries has added to the level of disease in some areas, and has been a continuing source of TB, although it is not clear whether immigration in recent years has contributed substantially more to TB than it has in the past (31). Growing numbers of inmates in correctional institutions, of residents in homeless shelters, and of patients with AIDS in health care facilities may also have contributed to rapid increases in TB in some areas. It is likely that a combination of many of these factors in the same populations produced the most volatile situation for TB.

Despite the multitude of social factors favoring its spread, most of which are not new, most TB cases are curable and preventable by traditional public health and medical approaches (see chapters 4 and 5). The withdrawal of public resources and the dismantling and defunding of community control programs credited with the earlier decline in the disease appear to have played a major role in the resurgence (31,45,240). Although the proportion of current cases that could have been prevented by surveillance and treatment is not known, the majority of them potentially could have been prevented. Moreover, the emergence of MDR-TB is a sensitive indicator of deficiencies in the process of ensuring treatment until cure, one of the main responsibilities of TB control programs.

Strategies to Prevent Tuberculous Infection and Active Disease | 4

There are many approaches to tuberculosis (TB) prevention, ranging from basic public health measures to technologically complex interventions. In the broadest sense, improvements in the standard of living, particularly less crowded housing and better health status overall, probably contributed the most to reducing the incidence of TB earlier this century and maintaining it since then at relatively low levels in the United States compared with many other countries. Over the past three decades, the development of effective medical treatment for TB has drastically reduced the period of infectivity in individuals with active disease and allowed for cure in the majority of cases treated (see chapter 5). Public health efforts to find cases of active TB, deliver curative treatment, investigate possible contacts of infectious cases, test them for infection, offer information about the disease, and deliver preventive treatment have become efficient means to break the chain of transmission (91). In hospitals, prisons, homeless shelters, and other congregate settings where infectious patients may be in close contact with others, infection control measures of various types are used to protect the uninfected from respiratory exposure to infectious individuals.

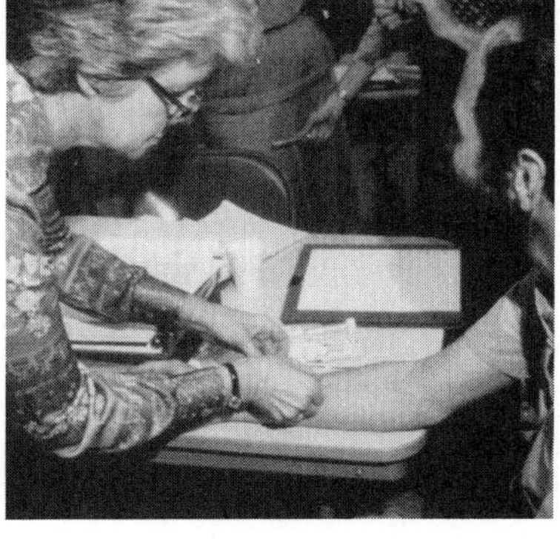

Once tuberculous infection occurs in an individual, measures can also be taken to lessen the chance that active disease will develop months or years later. Preventive treatment (after infection) and bacillus Calmette-Guérin (BCG) vaccination (before infection) are the two main approaches used to prevent the active TB.

This chapter examines three of these approaches—infection control measures to prevent transmission in institutional settings, preventive treatment, and BCG vaccination. The recent resurgence of TB, along with multidrug resistant-TB (MDR-TB) transmission and coinfection with human immunodeficiency virus (HIV), has brought some of the old issues in TB prevention to light and created new ones. Current issues and problems, along with developments in progress to improve each approach, are also summarized.

INFECTION CONTROL

In the past several years, a series of large outbreaks of MDR-TB in hospitals, prisons and other facilities have renewed concern about TB transmission and prompted debate over the need for and usefulness of various approaches to prevent further spread of infection (20,101,223, 348,350,352a). Thus far, more than 250 individuals contracted MDR-TB in these outbreaks, the majority of whom died within a few months of diagnosis. In nearly all cases, the outbreak strain was resistant to isoniazid (INH) and rifampin (RIF), the two most effective anti-tuberculous drugs. Some cases were resistant to seven drugs. Sixteen health-care workers (HCWs) and one prison guard also developed MDR-TB, seven of whom have died. Eighty percent of the patients, inmates, and staff who developed active disease in these outbreaks were known to be HIV-seropositive or otherwise immunocompromised (e.g., resulting from radiation treatment for cancer) (80,382). Epidemiologic investigations confirmed that the cases were acquired by airborne infection within the facilities.

At two of the hospitals, about a third of HCWs exposed to patients with MDR-TB were found to have been recently infected around the time of the outbreaks. At another hospital, more than 50 previously uninfected HCWs tested positive for tuberculous infection following exposure to hospitalized inmates with MDR-TB. Transmission of MDR-TB infection to HCWs in the other hospitals could not be determined because of a lack of comparative test results (324,382). While it is impossible to exclude the possibility that some of the HCWs may have acquired tuberculous infection outside of the hospital, it is assumed that most of the HCWs' infections occurring during the outbreak periods resulted from exposure to infectious patients without adequate infection control measures in place.

It has been suggested that medical housestaff, nurses, and other HCWs have recently experienced high rates of new TB infection (151), but recent data on rates of tuberculous infection among HCWs have not yet been published. Although tuberculous infection has long been recognized as an occupational hazard for HCWs, the magnitude of the risk of infection has not been well characterized in recent years because routine annual screening for tuberculous infection among most HCWs has been discontinued in many areas or is not collected systematically or is not reported publicly. Several surveys have reported higher rates of tuberculous infection among physicians and hospital personnel than the general population, though not all cases of infection could be identified as having been acquired through occupational, rather than community, exposure (15,109,234).

Some evidence indicates that HCWs in certain job categories are at higher risk of infection than other HCWs. A 1983 national survey comparing TB infection rates among physician trainees found that physicians training in pulmonary medicine had a greater risk of infection than similarly exposed physicians training in infectious disease (182). The higher risk was thought to be due in large part to the pulmonary physicians' likelihood of exposure to patients with pulmonary TB and involvement with certain invasive respiratory procedures (such as bronchoscopy and endotracheal intubation) that stimulate the patient's coughing reflex.

The Centers for Disease Control and Prevention (CDC) recommends that routine surveillance of HCWs by tuberculin skin testing be conducted to monitor for possible infection in health care facilities (359). The particular vulnerabilities of HIV-infected HCWs to occupational TB exposure has recently prompted CDC and others to examine that issue (22,214).

Two features clearly distinguish the recent outbreaks from those of the past: undiagnosed or inadequately treated MDR-TB as a potent source of infection, and heightened vulnerability of immunocompromised individuals to rapid development of active TB. The fact that these outbreaks occurred in facilities in different regions of the country suggests that the problem is not specific to certain hospitals or local populations, but is a broader issue affecting individuals with HIV, HCWs, prison staff, and the community at large. The potential exists for nosocomial (acquired within the hospital) transmission of TB in many urban areas, given increasing numbers of hospitalized, incarcerated, and homeless individuals with acquired immunodeficiency virus (AIDS), rising rates of TB in these populations, and inadequate infection control measures for preventing the spread of infection within the facilities (80,87). Transmission of drug-susceptible TB may also be occurring, although it is less likely that such clusters would be recognized since they would be indistinguishable from most other cases in the community.

Investigations of the outbreaks revealed a common set of problems and deficiencies that allowed the disease to spread unchecked (20,87,223). Failure or delay in diagnosing TB in patients and inmates was cited as a major factor. One reason for this was the often unusual clinical and radiographic presentation of TB in individuals with AIDS, which may obscure or complicate the diagnosis. Further, a "low index of suspicion" for TB among HCWs unaccustomed to seeing patients with the disease was cited for HCWs' failure to order appropriate diagnostic tests upon admission so that potentially infectious patients could be isolated until they were determined to be noninfectious. In addition, laboratory procedures caused additional delays in obtaining diagnoses, confirmation, and drug susceptibility results. In one hospital, for example, a median of 15 weeks elapsed between the time patients' specimens were obtained and the time results were available due (223), in large part, to the slow growth rate of the bacilli.

Failure to render MDR-TB patients noninfectious through adequate treatment was another major factor in the outbreaks. In many cases, prolonged periods of infectiousness occurred despite treatment, either because the specific type of resistance was not yet identified and ineffective drugs were prescribed, or because the few remaining drugs available to treat patients with multiple resistance were not effective. The latter undoubtedly applied to the cases in which resistance to seven drugs was documented, but even in cases resistant only to INH and RIF, successful outcomes are far more difficult to obtain (see chapter 5). Treatment failure then led to the persistence of symptoms (such as coughing), longer hospital stays, and a greater risk of transmission of infection to others.

Despite these serious problems, it is likely that transmission of tuberculous infection within the facilities could have been substantially reduced, if not totally prevented, by better use of recommended infection control measures. Investigations of the outbreaks revealed a number of common problems in applying and maintaining infection control measures. In various ways, respiratory isolation of infectious patients was either not achieved (i.e., the facility was not designed to handle infectious TB patients) or isolation was not consistently maintained. For example, ventilation systems permitted air from the patients' rooms to mix with surrounding areas rather than providing negative pressure relative to the corridors and other rooms. Often these systems recirculated the air within the facility rather than exhausting it directly to the outside. Patients who were in respiratory isolation sometimes left their rooms to walk to bathrooms down the hall, or their doors were left open to the corridors. Also noted was an insufficient number of properly equipped isolation rooms to accommodate the number of patients with suspected or confirmed TB. In some cases, isolation precautions were

Box 4-A—Summary of Recommendations for Preventing the Transmission of Tuberculosis in Healthcare Settings, 1992

Early identification and treatment of persons with active tuberculosis

- Maintain a high index of suspicion for TB to identify cases rapidly.
- Promptly initiate effective multidrug anti-TB therapy based on clinical and drug-resistance surveillance data.

Prevention of spread of infectious droplet nuclei by source control methods and by reduction of microbial contamination of indoor air

- Initiate acid-fast bacilli (AFB) isolation precautions immediately for all patients who are suspected or confirmed to have active TB and who may be infectious. AFB isolation precautions include use of a private room with negative pressure in relation to surrounding areas and a minimum of six air exchanges per hour. Air from the room should be exhausted directly to the outside. Use of ultraviolet lamps and/or high-efficiency particulate air filters to supplement ventilation may be considered.
- Persons entering the AFB isolation room should use disposable particulate respirators that fit snugly around the face.
- Continue AFB isolation precautions until there is clinical evidence of reduced infectiousness (i.e., cough has substantially decreased, and the number of organisms on sequential sputum smears is decreasing). If drug resistance is suspected or confirmed, continue AFB precautions until the sputum smear is negative for AFB.
- Use special precautions during cough-inducing procedures.

Surveillance for TB transmission

- Maintain surveillance for TB infection among health-care workers (HCWs) by routine, periodic tuberculin skin testing. Recommend appropriate preventive therapy for HCWs when indicated.
- Maintain surveillance for TB cases among patients and HCWs.
- Promptly initiate contact investigation procedures among HCWs, patients, and visitors exposed to an untreated, or inefficiently treated, infectious TB patient for whom appropriate AFB procedures are not in place. Recommend appropriate therapy or preventive therapy for contacts with disease or TB infection without current disease. Therapeutic regimens should be chosen based on the clinical history and local drug-resistance surveillance data.

SOURCE: U.S. Department of Health and Human Services, Public Health Service, Centers for Disease Control and Prevention, 1992.

discontinued prematurely, while patients were still infectious.

A number of specific circumstances further increased the probability that infection would be spread. Most notably, two commonly used procedures—pentamidine aerosol treatment for patients with AIDS and sputum induction to collect samples for TB diagnosis—elicit forceful coughing, propelling infectious particles into the air unless contained in specially-designed booths (52). Both procedures have previously been associated with increased transmission of tuberculous infection in health care facilities (345).

Infection Control Measures

For many years, the merits and drawbacks of various infection control strategies have been debated. CDC recently updated and expanded its comprehensive guidelines for preventing transmission of tuberculous infection within hospitals and other facilities (359). These guidelines (which are now undergoing further revision) call for stricter application of a broad range of strategies (see box 4-A), some of which involve relatively simple modifications of procedures, while others involve the incorporation of sophisticated and expensive technologies. It is believed that such

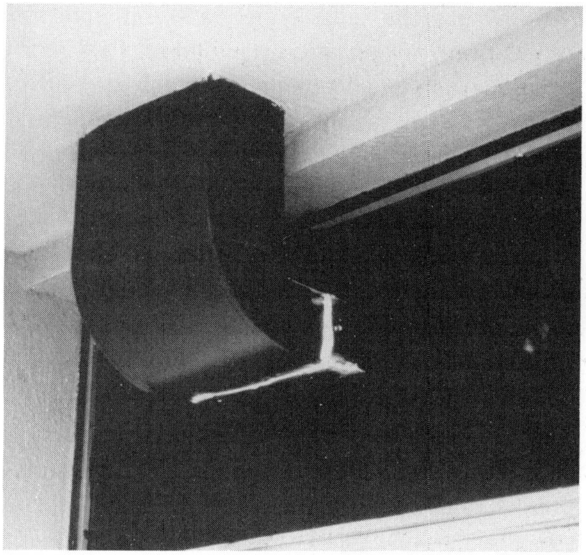

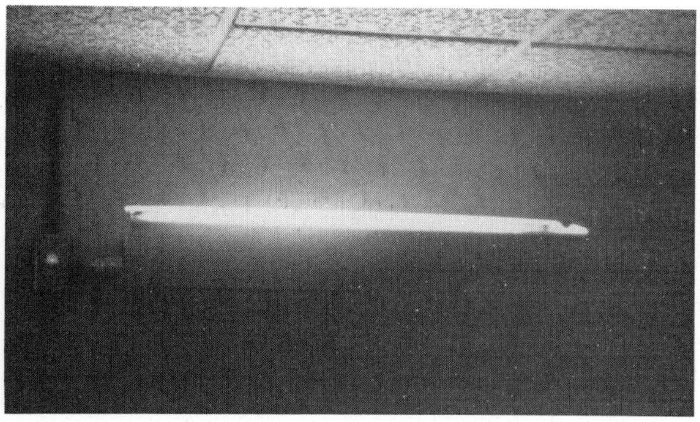

CDC and NYU MEDICAL CENTER

Adequate ventilation and ultraviolet-B light can both decrease the likelihood of acquiring TB infection. Here an ultraviolet light (above) and an exhaust fan (left) have been added to some hospital rooms housing patients with infectious TB to help control the spread of the disease.

measures have not yet been widely adopted by health care facilities (254).

CDC's guidelines emphasized a "hierarchy of controls," emphasizing first the implementation of source control and administrative measures to reduce or eliminate the production of infectious particles or confine them to the patient where they originate—e.g., rapid identification of infectious patients, prompt initiation of treatment, respiratory isolation of infectious patients, and instructing patients to wear masks or cover their mouths when they cough. These measures are generally considered to comprise the first and most important line of defense against transmission of tuberculous infection in institutional settings (21).

Additional measures to be used after the previous and administrative ones are in place included environmental controls for eliminating infectious particles after they have been released into the air (such as redirecting air flow and filtering or irradiating the air to remove infectious particles). Adequate ventilation generally includes directional air flow into isolation rooms from adjacent areas, air filtration, and direct exhaust of air to the outside. A minimum of six air exchanges per hour in isolation rooms is specified in CDC's guidelines. Such measures are not necessarily easy to implement in modern facilities that are designed to recirculate air for energy conservation or in older buildings with no central air circulation. New devices are currently in development to filter and recirculate air within individual rooms, although their usefulness is far from demonstrated (205).

Disinfection of air with ultraviolet (UV) light sources has also been advocated (252). It is known from experimental data that tubercle bacilli are readily killed by UV-C irradiation (ultraviolet radiation of a shorter wavelength than UV-B present in sunlight), but data on efficacy in killing airborne tubercle bacilli under actual use conditions are lacking. Relevant variables include the intensity of the radiation, duration of contact, and humidity of the air. The minimum effective dose is unknown. Special fixtures have been developed for overhead installation but precise recommendations for their design and installation have not yet been developed. Such devices could be particularly appropriate where adequate ventilation and air filtration are impossible to attain. At present, a number of practical issues limit the effectiveness and application of such lights under different conditions; however, modifications are likely to be made to permit wider use. These lights pose a potential risk for temporary but painful photokeratitis (inflammation of the cornea of the eye), which can result from exposure to high-intensity UV-C light (206), so care needs to be taken to prevent direct exposure. The safety of properly designed UV-C lights on patients and HCWs under actual conditions has not been studied systematically. Anecdotal reports point to success with UV systems in some high-risk settings (151).

The final type of measure discussed in CDC's guidelines on infection control was personal protection devices, such as particulate respirators. Standard surgical face masks probably do not protect adequately against TB infection because they allow inhalation of airborne particles around the outside of the mask, although there is no evidence that they have failed to protect against infection. Masks designed to fit tightly around the nose and mouth (disposable particulate respirators) are believed to provide at least some protection against tubercle bacilli, but again, relevant data are lacking.

One of the most controversial aspects of infection control concerns the use of "powered air purification respirators" (PAPRs), which are powered, halfmask respirators equipped with high-efficiency particulate filters. They are commonly used in industrial settings to protect workers from toxic fumes and other substances. The National Institute for Occupational Safety and Health (NIOSH), an agency within CDC, proposed in a recent report to the Occupational Safety and Health Administration, that PAPRs be used to protect high-risk HCWs from occupational exposure to tuberculous infection (371); NIOSH is mandated by the Occupational Safety and Health Act of 1970 to "formulate science-based assessments of risk and preventive recommendations, which, if implemented, would assure that no worker develops illness as a consequence of exposure at work." Many experts have argued that such devices are unnecessary, uncomfortable, and impractical in clinical situations (151,328).

To review the underlying data and practical implications of this recommendation, CDC convened a group of experts in TB infection control, biosafety, occupational safety and health, and representatives of labor groups and other organizations. William L. Roper, CDC's director, concluded from the meeting that current evidence was inadequate to determine the effectiveness of such respirators in protecting HCWs from nosocomial transmission and that their routine use in health-care settings was not recommended (254).

There appear to be no clinical studies evaluating the efficacy of any of the various infection control measures to exist in preventing transmission of tuberculous infection (or other airborne infections). One reason for this is the difficulty of studying effects of single interventions in a clinical setting. Accordingly, precise judgments cannot yet be made about the efficacy or cost-effectiveness of the various measures. It is believed, however, that combinations of measures taken to improve infection control were responsible for the cessation of some of the outbreaks (e.g., in a Miami hospital) (219), the most important measure being rapid diagnosis and isolation of infectious patients. Nevertheless, data on the clinical efficacy, efficiency, and feasibility of the various measures will be needed in the long run to help guide these decisions.

In the short term, decisions about the necessity and appropriateness of individual measures in a given site will probably be determined largely by the prevalence of TB in that resident population, available resources, and the physical characteristics of each facility that influence the risk of transmission and the applicability of different interventions. Different combinations of interventions would be appropriate for different settings (see boxes 4-B through 4-D), e.g., acute care hospitals, prisons, HIV clinics, and homeless shelters. Infection control experts have recently recommended that such decisions be based on an individualized risk assessment for each local area, rather than on a universal set of requirements for both high- and low-prevalence areas (21).

Box 4-B—Changes in Infection Control Measures at Bellevue Hospital, New York City

Bellevue Hospital, one of New York City's largest municipal hospitals, admits more than 400 patients with active TB per year to its 1,232-bed facility. To protect against transmission of tuberculous infection within the hospital, extensive changes have recently been made in its infection control capabilities and procedures.

In addition to standard ventilation, which provides two fresh air exchanges per hour in each room, Bellevue's isolation and bronchoscopy rooms each have a window exhaust fan that allows four additional air exchanges per hour, with air expelled directly outside through a high-efficiency particulator air filter. This ventilation system is designed to create negative air flow relative to the corridor.

Each room also has been fitted with an air filtration system that recirculates air (at the rate of eight room volumes per hour) through a prefilter in tandem with a high-efficiency particulator air (HEPA) filter. This system is designed both to trap and remove airborne tubercle bacilli and also to facilitate mixing of the air, which enhances the bactericidal activity of ultraviolet lights.

The cost of these ventilation changes is estimated at $10,000 per isolation room.

Ultraviolet (UV) light fixtures have also been installed in each respiratory isolation room and in some of the common areas where patients with active TB are likely to be present, including waiting and examination areas, bronchoscopy rooms, radiology areas, and chest clinics. Each isolation room has two 30-watt UV fixtures, mounted on the wall above eye level to provide UV light for up to 200 square feet of floor space.

All hospital staff entering respiratory isolation rooms are required to wear a dust-mist particulate respirator. Health care workers performing certain high-risk procedures on patients with active TB, such as sputum induction, aerosolized pentamidine administration, and endotracheal intubation and suctioning, are required to wear a particulate respirator. Patients with active TB are required to wear masks only when outside of their isolation rooms.

SOURCE: W. Rom, Director and Professor, Department of Medicine, Division of Pulmonary and Critical Care Medicine, New York University Medical Center, New York, NY, personal communication, June 1993.

TUBERCULIN SKIN TESTING AND PREVENTIVE TREATMENT

Since the 1950s, when the anti-TB drug isoniazid (INH) was introduced and first evaluated for efficacy in treating active TB (see chapter 5), it has also been possible to use this drug for the treatment of tuberculous infection to prevent subsequent development of the active disease. A number of clinical trials aimed at evaluating the efficacy of INH as a preventive treatment have shown over 90 percent effectiveness afforded by completion of 12 months of INH preventive treatment (IPT) among individuals with tuberculous infection caused by INH-susceptible bacilli (64,113). Unless reinfection occurs later in life (generally unlikely in most U.S. populations), the benefits of IPT are presumed to be lifelong (113,131). IPT would not be expected to benefit individuals infected with INH-resistant tubercle bacilli.

Not all individuals with tuberculous infection are equally likely to develop active TB. Some develop it within a year or two after infection, while others harbor the infection for decades before becoming sick; most never develop the disease at all (249,300). The reasons for these differences are largely unknown, although some specific risk factors associated with a greater likelihood of progression have been identified. From a public health standpoint, the most important of these is HIV infection.

Public health efforts to prevent TB concentrate, for practical and economic reasons, on screening for tuberculous infection where it most likely is to be found—in identifiable high-risk groups (see tables 4-1 and 4-2). In total, an estimated 10 to 15 million individuals in the United States have

Box 4-C—Infection Control Measures at Cook County Hospital, Chicago

Cook County Hospital (CCH), a 950-bed municipal hospital on Chicago's near-west side, was built in 1910. Its physical plant is antiquated: 30-bed open wards still exist, heating is provided by radiators, and there is no air conditioning. Each year, approximately one-quarter of Chicago's newly diagnosed TB patients are diagnosed at CCH (168 patients in 1991); over 300 with active TB were admitted to CCH in 1990. A long-suspected problem with occupational exposure to TB was recently documented in a study of tuberculin skin test conversions among CCH staff physicians; purified protein derivative conversions after 1 year of clinical work at CCH were noted among 46 percent of housestaff training in internal medicine, compared with 5 percent of other physician trainees (in emergency medicine, family practice, obstetrics/gynecology, pediatrics, and radiology).

To address the problem, CCH implemented infection control measures according to the Centers for Disease Control and Prevention's 1990 guidelines, with adjustment for the hospital's physical plant, available resources, and patient care and health-care workers (HCWs) concerns. All 51 single rooms with bathrooms were outfitted with fans that expel room air outside at a rate sufficient to provide 6 or more air changes per hour and negative air flow relative to the halls, and with a ultraviolet light. Common areas of the hospital where occupational exposure might occur, including the pulmonary function test laboratory and a labor and delivery room, were also outfitted with fans and UV lights.

A triage protocol was developed for CCH's emergency room and walk-in clinics to speed identification and isolation of patients with known or suspected TB. Sputum induction booths were installed in the emergency room, HIV clinic, and the admitting ward. Emergency room laboratory personnel were trained and equipped to perform sputum smear examinations on site to avoid sending specimens out to the microbiology laboratory for processing. Admitting procedures were changed so that patients with active TB could be admitted directly to isolation rooms without going through the common admitting ward.

Surgical masks were replaced with particulate respirators for all HCWs and visitors entering respiratory isolation rooms. HCWs were given training sessions on nosocomial transmission of TB and measures to protect themselves from infection. Two nurses were hired to serve as a roving employee health service team to offer tuberculin skin testing to HCWs at their worksites within the hospital.

The total cost of ventilation changes, UV lights, particulate respirators, and additional personnel was estimated at $350,000 in 1992, with ongoing annual costs of approximately $100,000. Since these infection control measures have been implemented, tuberculin skin test conversions among CCH housestaff have dropped from 15 percent per year in 1991 to around 6 percent in 1992 and 1993. The tuberculin skin testing program is currently reaching about half of the hospital's HCWs at risk for occupational exposure to TB.

SOURCE: City of Chicago, Department of Health, "Tuberculosis Morbidity and Mortality Report. 1991," Tuberculosis Control Program, City of Chicago, Chicago, IL, August 25, 1992; L. Cocchiarella, R. Cohen, and S. Muzaffar, "PPD Conversion Among Housestaff in a Public Hospital" (abstract) *American Review of Respiratory Diseases* 145(4):(Suppl) A102, 1992; Rebecca M. Wurtz, Director, Section of Epidemiology, Department of Infectious Diseases, Cook County Hospital, Chicago, IL, personal communication, June 1993.

tuberculous infection (357). However, the prevalence of tuberculous infection in specific populations and geographic areas is unknown, since the practice of regular screening among children and adults was abandoned during the 1970s and 1980s. No national surveys of tuberculous infection have been conducted in the United States in over 20 years. Recent small surveys of children in certain urban areas, however, have shown high rates of infection, particularly among foreign-born children (307). At present, only three States (Indiana, Missouri, and Kentucky) require reporting of tuberculin skin test results in children under six (307).

The medical community and public health officials in the United States have long advocated the policy of selective use of IPT. Recent increases in the incidence of TB in communities with high rates of HIV, along with evidence of rapid progression to active TB among those with

Box 4-D—Infection Control Measures at the Rikers Island Correctional System, New York City

The tuberculosis case rate in the New York City correctional system is close to 600 cases per 100,000 population—three times the highest case rate in the general population of New York City. Montefiore Medical Center, a private not-for-profit hospital in the Bronx, in a tripartite agreement with the New York City Department of Health and Correction, provides comprehensive health services to the 14,000 men and women incarcerated on Rikers Island Correctional Complex. The Montefiore Rikers Island Health Services has worked closely with both agencies over the past few years on the implementation of infection control measures in the jails to curb the increase in TB. Currently, 125 individuals are being treated for active tuberculosis. The TB control program is challenged by the high turnover of the population, the short average length of stay of 59 days (with half of new admissions discharged from the system within a week), and the rapid transfer of inmates between different facilities. The creation of a respiratory isolation area, the development of a computerized tracking system, and the increasing ability of the Department of Correction to locate prisoners within the system have facilitated their ability to treat patients on TB medications.

To complement a TB control system that includes systematic screening, diagnosis, treatment, and contact tracing among inmates, Rikers Island has instituted a series of environmental changes in its facilities to help stop the spread of the disease.

In May 1992, the Department of Correction in conjunction with the Department of Health, Montefiore Rikers Island Health Services and other city agencies opened its first 42 isolation beds. There are 140 such respiratory isolation beds. Tent structures erected for housing of inmates were retrofitted to achieve levels of respiratory isolation that exceed all State, city, and CDC guidelines. Each room has approximately 10 to 12 air exchanges per hour, vents air to the outside, and has an anteroom with positive pressure. The corridor has approximately 18 air exchanges per hour. An extensive computer system monitors any cessation of negative pressure or other malfunction and makes appropriate adjustments or notifications.

All patients with suspected or confirmed TB are placed in respiratory isolation until TB is ruled out or until they are no longer infectious and have been evaluated for placement in the general jail population.

The facility has medical and nursing personnel 24 hours a day. Mental health services are provided daily for the many patients who also suffer from mental illness or who have mental health crises triggered by their isolation or adverse side effects from their medications. An estimated 60 percent are dually diagnosed with HIV infection and have complicated medical conditions. TB patients wear surgical masks when outside of their rooms; the more confining particulate respiratory masks may impair their breathing.

Upon release from jail, all patients receiving treatment for TB receive an appointment card that lists their medications, diagnosis, and the location of a community-based clinic that will provide directly observed therapy (DOT) to ensure continuity of treatment. These clinics include the Department of Health Chest Clinics and private providers who provide DOT through the State Medicaid program.

Due to the high prevalence of TB in correctional settings, all Montefiore employees receive a purified protein derivative (PPD) skin test every 6 months. Employees working in high-risk areas receive a PPD skin test every 3 months. Rikers Island has developed a computerized tracking system that automatically generates lists of those employees due for a skin test and documents the results of those tests. Rikers Island also provides education about TB for non-clinical staff including the appropriate use of particulate respirator masks worn in the presence of suspected or confirmed TB patients.

SOURCE: L. Richmond, Assistant to the Director, Montefiore Rikers Island Health Services, Montefiore Medical Center, The University Hospital for the Albert Einstein College of Medicine, New York, NY, personal communication, 1993.

Table 4-1—Risk Factors for Tuberculous Infection

- Close contact with infectious tuberculosis cases (e.g., in the same household).
- Immigration from areas of high TB prevalence (i.e., parts of Asia, Africa, Latin America, and the Caribbean).
- Low-income status (including homeless people and migrant farm workers).
- Racial or ethnic minority (including African American, Hispanic, Native American).
- Substance abuse (especially alcohol and intravenous drugs).
- Residence in correctional institution, nursing home, mental institution, or other long-term care facility.

SOURCES: A.B. Bloch, H.L. Rieder, G.D. Kelly, et al., "The Epidemiology of Tuberculosis in the United States. Implications for Diagnosis and Treatment," *Clinics in Chest Medicine* 10(3):297-313, 1989; U.S. Department of Health and Human Services, Public Health Service, U.S. Centers for Disease Control and Prevention, "Screening for Tuberculosis and Tuberculous Infection in High-Risk Populations. Recommendations of the Advisory Committee for Elimination of Tuberculosis," *Morbidity and Mortality Weekly Report* 39(RR-8):1-12, 1990.

both HIV and tuberculous infection (278,290), have prompted renewed calls for expanding the use of IPT. Even in many developing countries, where IPT has never been feasible because of the sheer number of people involved and the lack of adequate resources to deliver treatment (387), the escalating cost of treating the enormous number of active cases expected in the near future now makes IPT appear to be a relatively less expensive option for controlling TB (76,202,203).

For several decades, it has been theoretically possible to prevent the majority of new TB cases in the United States with the available diagnostic and preventive treatment methods. As TB has receded from the general population and become more concentrated among particular populations defined by ethnicity, race, geography, and age (see chapter 3), such targeted efforts at prevention should have become more feasible (28). However, because of limited resources available to TB control programs, controversies about adverse effects of IPT, problems with access to medical care, difficulties in ensuring completion of lengthy treatment regimens, among other reasons, IPT has not been widely applied, even in the high-risk populations for which it is most highly recommended (2,17,115,381). According to national data collected by CDC, fewer than half of all individuals with tuberculous infection identified by TB control programs through contact investigation receive an adequate course of preventive treatment (111).

Notable efforts have recently been made in some areas to overcome these obstacles, as in a program to offer IPT under direct observation to residents of a Seattle homeless shelter (208). In a nationwide effort involving 25 sites, CDC recently funded a project to evaluate the feasibility of onsite screening for tuberculous infection and for provision of IPT for clients at drug-treatment centers and inmates at Federal and State correctional facilities (355). Among the more than 38,000 individuals tested, 16 percent were found to have tuberculous infection (13 percent of drug-treatment clients and 25 percent of inmates); 66 percent of the infected drug-treatment clients, compared with 94 percent of infected inmates, subsequently completed IPT. Although the project showed that screening could be successfully conducted at these sites, ensuring completion of

Table 4-2—Risk Factors for Progression from Tuberculous Infection to Active TB

- Symptoms suggestive of TB.
- HIV infection.
- Previously untreated TB.
- Underweight (at least 10 percent below ideal body weight).
- Medical conditions known to increase the risk of TB once infected (e.g., silicosis, diabetes mellitus, chronic renal failure, gastrectomy, some forms of cancer, treatment with immunosuppressive agents).
- Extremely young age.

SOURCES: A.B. Bloch, H.L. Rieder, G.D. Kelly, et al., "The Epidemiology of Tuberculosis in the United States. Implications for Diagnosis and Treatment," *Clinics in Chest Medicine* 10(3):297-313, 1989; U.S. Department of Health and Human Services, Centers for Disease Control, "Screening for Tuberculosis and Tuberculous Infection in High-Risk Populations. Recommendations of the Advisory Committee for Elimination of Tuberculosis," *Morbidity and Mortality Weekly Report* 39(RR-8):1-12, 1990.

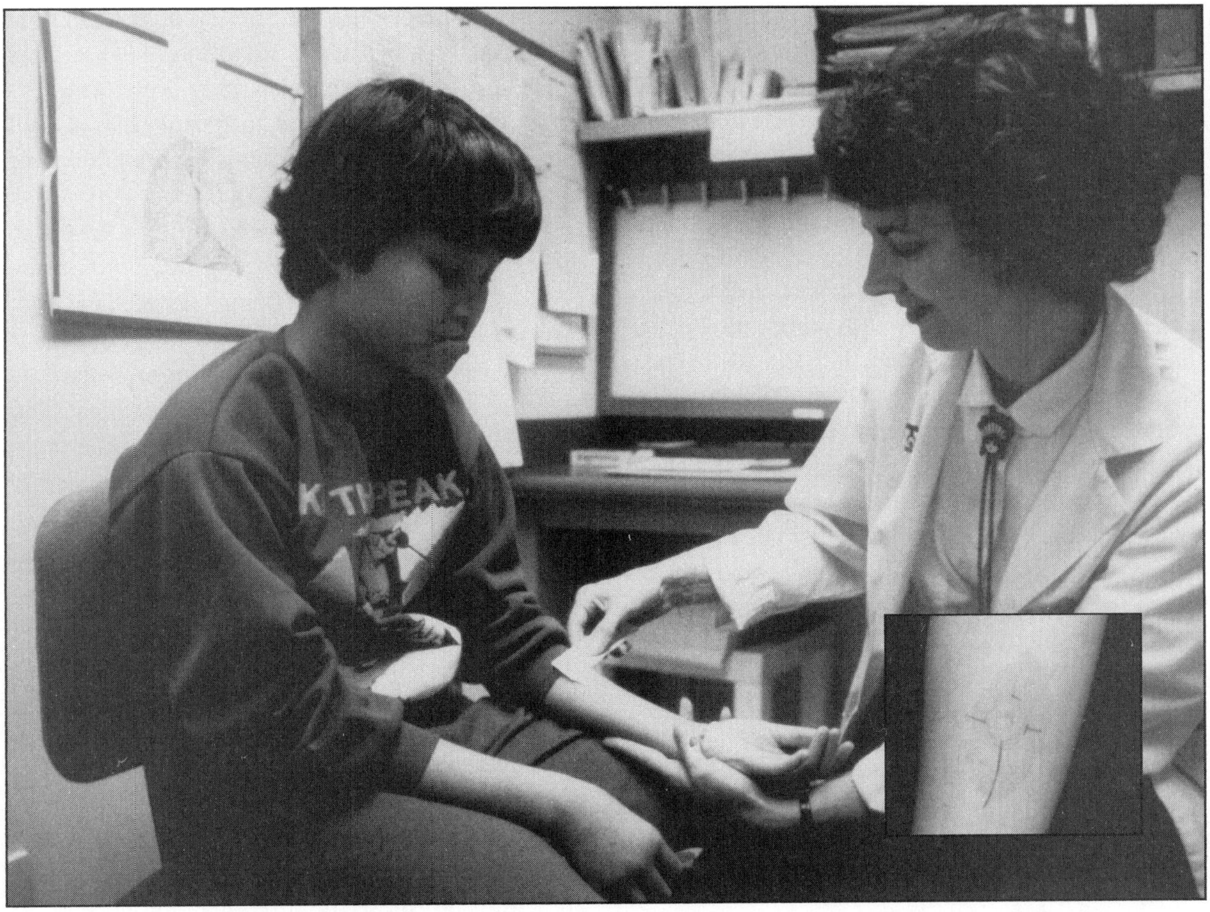

CENTERS FOR DISEASE CONTROL AND PREVENTION

The TB skin test, in which a purified protein derivative is injected under the skin, produces a reaction like the one on the right in about 95 percent of immunocompetent individuals infected with the bacilli that cause TB. The test detects infection in a much smaller percentage of people with HIV or other types of immunosupression.

IPT still posed substantial difficulties in the drug-treatment setting.

The following section briefly describes the available methods for identifying individuals with tuberculous infection and for preventing the development of active TB.

Identifying Individuals with Tuberculous Infection

At present, methods for directly detecting the presence of tubercle bacilli in the body (see chapter 5) are applicable only for those with active TB, which normally creates a large number of bacilli in the body. By contrast, latent tuberculous infection creates much smaller populations of bacilli in the body and is not directly detectable with current microbiologic methods (isolating, culturing, and identifying populations of organisms) or histologic methods (staining a sample containing bacilli and visually identifying them under the microscope).

The preferred means to identify individuals with tuberculous infection is the tuberculin skin test, developed in the 1890s and still in widespread use (268). As an indirect approach, the tuberculin skin test is designed to show a type of immune response (a delayed-type hypersensitivity (DTH) response mediated by T-lymphocytes) to tuberculin, proteins derived from a culture of tubercle bacilli (see chapter 2). Normally, the immune system of individuals infected with tubercle bacilli will be sensitized to tuberculin and will react (within 48 to 72 hours) to the test substance, as shown by a small raised area (usually greater than 10 mm) in the skin on the arm where the tuberculin is given. Individuals without previous exposure to tubercle bacilli should show no reaction on the skin to the test substance, unless they have had BCG vaccination or have been infected with nontuberculous mycobacteria.

For various reasons, responses to the tuberculin skin test are not "all or nothing" small reactions (5 to 10 mm) could mean infection in some and no infection in others. The test results must be interpreted in light of the individual's risk for TB infection, previous BCG vaccination, age, immunocompetence, and exposure to mycobacteria other than tubercle bacilli, among other factors. A complex system for interpreting the test result for each individual based on risk factors, medical history, and size of the skin reaction has been developed (7,357).

In healthy individuals, the test has about 95 percent sensitivity and variable specificity (18,268). In individuals who are infected with HIV or who are acutely ill (with various viral infections, or, ironically, acute or overwhelming TB), its sensitivity is consistently lower or nonexistent; the test cannot be used in these circumstances to exclude the possibility of tuberculous infection (18,361). For practical purposes, negative results in individuals with late stage HIV are uninterpretable (126,143,361). Unless the tuberculin skin test is given early in the course of HIV infection, detection of true infection is much less likely, and thereby reduces the efficacy and usefulness of preventive treatment. CDC recommends that since HIV-infected individuals with tuberculous infection are at such high risk for developing active TB, IPT should be given to those with HIV who show small skin test reactions of 5 mm or more or to those who are anergic and who are at high risk for tuberculous infection (344). Others have argued for bypassing skin tests in HIV-infected individuals and offering IPT to all individuals with AIDS where the prevalence of tuberculous infection is high (165).

The accuracy of the tuberculin skin test also varies with the prevalence of tuberculous infection in the population being tested. In high prevalence groups (more than 25 percent infected), such as immigrants from high-prevalence areas of Asia, Africa, or Latin America, and recent, close contacts of active cases, tuberculin screening is generally considered to be informative and reliable. For many other populations, prevalence data are likely to be unavailable, so unless an individual is known to have been exposed to an infectious case or has other risk factors, interpreting the results of tuberculin skin tests is problematic. In very low-risk populations (prevalence of tuberulous infection less than 1 percent), such as the general U.S. adult population or, in many areas of the country, children entering school, the vast majority of positive results are likely to be falsely positive (18). Screening in these populations could lead to unnecessary isolation, testing, and treatment based on an erroneous presumption of TB. For that reason, tuberculin skin testing in low-risk populations is generally discouraged.

Limitations of the current tuberculin skin test may become increasingly apparent as screening is expanded to include more individuals with HIV, including homeless individuals, foreign-born individuals, and others. Improvements in the diagnostic capabilities for detecting infection are clearly needed. Specifically, a test that can be read without a long waiting period would be particularly useful in institutional settings where individuals may be difficult to locate several days later (e.g., jails and homeless shelters). A test that accurately and directly detects the infection and identifies the drug resistance pattern of the bacilli without depending on adequate immune responses to the infection would be essential for use in HIV-infected populations.

Isoniazid Preventive Treatment

The purpose of preventive treatment is to eliminate the living tubercle bacilli in the body, thereby reducing the risk of subsequent disease. These bacilli may be growing slowly, intermittently, or not at all. A treatment regimen based on the use of a single antibiotic drug for a long period of time (6 to 12 months) is necessary to substantially reduce the risk of subsequent disease. The chance of creating drug resistance in the process is considered low, since there are so few bacilli to begin with and only a remote chance that any drug-resistant ones are present. In the absence of disease, distinguishing infection with drug-resistant bacilli from infection with drug-sensitive bacilli is impossible with current diagnostic methods. Epidemiologic investigations could suggest the likelihood of drug resistance, and assist with the choice of drugs to be used in preventive treatment (13).

So far, INH is the only drug evaluated in human studies for efficacy in preventing progression of tuberculous infection. The American Thoracic Society, medical section of the American Lung Association, recommendations state that when INH cannot be tolerated, or if infection with INH-resistant bacilli is suspected, rifampin (RIF) can be used for preventive treatment in high-risk individuals (6,13). Data on the efficacy of RIF and other antibiotics in preventing TB are currently lacking. Animal data suggest that shorter regimens, e.g., 2 months of twice-weekly treatment, using RIF and pyrazinamide (PZA), are good candidates for study (150), and several clinical trials are in progress (e.g., in Haiti) (60). A recent placebo-controlled trial conducted in Hong Kong found that 3 months of RIF was as effective as 6 months of INH in preventing the onset of TB (138). It is not yet known whether regimens consisting of RIF and PZA for 2 months' duration will replace longer courses of INH for preventive treatment (131). The effectiveness and costs of these new approaches have not been examined in detail.

The efficacy of INH in preventing TB is well established through a series of randomized controlled trials involving more than 125,000 subjects. Results indicate that IPT can reduce the risk of active TB among adults with tuberculous infection by as much as 90 percent in those who complete a full course of treatment and by about 50 to 60 percent if those who don't complete treatment are included in the analysis (13,97,148). In children, the reduction in risk approaches 100 percent (142).

The efficacy of preventive treatment for TB in HIV-infected individuals with tuberculous infection has not yet been reported from controlled trials (although such trials are in progress in Zambia (383) and elsewhere) (202). Preliminary results from one of the trials suggest that a 12-month course of IPT can lead to a 89 percent reduction in TB among HIV-infected individuals compared with a placebo. In its 1989 report on TB and HIV infection, CDC recommended that HIV-infected individuals with tuberculous infection should be offered IPT for a 12-month period, based on evidence of effectiveness in HIV-negative populations and observations of success with curative treatment for active TB in HIV-infected patients (344). Subsequent observational data supported the use of IPT in HIV-infected patients (279). The National Institute of Allergy and Infectious Diseases (NIAID) is currently supporting two clinical trials to evaluate the efficacy of IPT in HIV-infected individuals (96).

One of the main reasons to evaluate alternatives to INH in preventive treatment is to avoid the risk of rare, though serious, adverse effects from the use of INH (in individuals who are not sick with TB and not infectious to others). The major concern is with toxic effects on the liver and potentially fatal hepatitis. Although the drug is well tolerated in most cases, particularly in children, between 2 to 3 percent of adults over age 50 develop liver inflammation (which can lead to

Table 4-3—Criteria for Determining Need for Preventive Therapy for Persons with Positive Tuberculin Reactions, by Category and Age Group

	Age group (years)	
Category	<35	≥35
With risk factor[a]	Treat at all ages if reaction to 5TU PPD ≥10 mm (or ≥5 mm and patient is recent contact, HIV-infected, *or* has radiographic evidence of old TB).	Treat at all ages if reaction to 5TU PPD ≥10 mm (or ≥5 mm and patient is recent contact, HIV-infected, *or* has radiographic evidence of old TB).
No risk factor. High-incidence group[b]	Treat if PPD ≥10mm.	Do not treat.
No risk factor. Low-incidence group	Treat if PPD ≥15mm[c].	Do not treat.

[a] Risk factors include HIV infection, recent contact with infectious person, recent skin-test conversion, abnormal chest radiograph, intravenous drug abuse, and certain medical risk factors (see text).

[b] High-incidence groups include foreign-born persons, medically underserved low-income populations, and residents of long-term care facilities.

[c] Lower or higher cut points may be used for identifying positive reactions, depending on the relative prevalence of *Myobacterium tuberculosis* infection and nonspecific cross-reactivity in the population.

KEY: PPD = purified protein derivative; TU = tuberculin unit.

SOURCE: U.S. Department of Health and Human Services, Public Health Service, Centers for Disease Control and Prevention, "The Use of Preventive Therapy for Tuberculous Infection in U.S. Recommendations of the Advisory Committee for Elimination of Tuberculosis," *Morbidity and Mortality Review* 29(RR-8):6-8, 1990.

hepatitis if the drug is not stopped as soon as serum tests indicate the condition). A recent review of available case reports of fatal hepatitis possibly associated with INH indicates that such cases seem to be decreasing in frequency since the early 1970s (possibly because of more limited use of IPT, but also because of better biochemical and clinical monitoring of patients on IPT). However, such cases are still occurring, especially among African American and Hispanic women (294). The postpartum period may be an especially high-risk time. Factors that increase the risk of INH-associated hepatitis may include alcohol or drug abuse, previous hepatitis, or simultaneous use of hepatotoxic drugs. The magnitude of the risk, and the specific factors contributing to it, are still largely unknown.

If IPT were harmless, there would be little controversy about offering it to virtually anyone with tuberculous infection would exist. Since it is not, disputes over balancing the risks and benefits in low-risk populations are difficult to resolve (65). A series of decision analyses comparing the risks of INH-induced hepatotoxicity with the benefits of preventing TB in low-risk populations have been published, with conflicting results (102,164,220,256,292,320). CDC developed criteria for determining how the use of IPT could be limited to minimize the risks of hepatoxicity and benefit those at highest risk. These criteria recommend avoiding use of IPT in low-risk populations (see table 4-3). Until alternative regimens with drugs posing fewer and less serious side effects are available, IPT will likely be limited to these high-risk groups.

BCG VACCINATION

Since the early 1950s, the World Health Organization (WHO) has advocated widespread vaccination with BCG as a preventive measure against TB. At present, over 70 percent of children worldwide are given BCG in infancy or childhood (386). Recommendations for vaccination schedules differ widely among countries, ranging from a single dose at birth (recommended by the WHO Expanded Programme on Immunization) to a single dose at age 13 (United Kingdom policy) to repeated vaccinations throughout childhood (as in many Eastern European countries). BCG vaccination is compulsory in 64 countries and officially recommended in 118 others (58). As a result of these policies, BCG has become the most widely used vaccine in the world, with more than 3 billion doses administered over the past 40 years (98).

Despite its widespread acceptance and longstanding use, controversy persists concerning the variation and lack of predictability in BCG's protective efficacy against TB in different populations. In part because of questions about its efficacy and low expected utility in populations in which the rate of transmission of TB is relatively low, BCG vaccination has never been applied on a national basis in the United States. As of 1988, when CDC's Immunization Practices Advisory Committee and Advisory Committee for Elimination of TB last issued recommendations on BCG use, a very circumscribed role for BCG vaccines was specified (343). Reexamination of the policy, along with renewed calls for development of an improved vaccine, are likely in the near future as CDC and others consider options for containing the current spread of TB.

This section briefly summarizes BCG's nature, intended effects, efficacy and safety, overall impact, and policy issues concerning its role in TB control efforts in the United States. Because of the enormity of the international literature on this subject dating back to the 1920s, only a brief overview is possible in the context of this report.

The Nature and Rationale for BCG Vaccines

BCG refers to several strains of *Mycobacterium bovis* derived from the original strain, which was produced about 70 years ago in France by Albert Calmette and Camille Guérin at the Pasteur Institute. Using a virulent strain of *Mycobacterium bovis*, the bacillus that causes tuberculosis in cattle and in humans,[1] Calmette and Guérin produced an attenuated bacterial isolate (a strain of tubercle bacilli unable to cause TB). Their product, consisting of a liquid preparation of live bacilli, was first used as an anti-TB vaccine in French subjects (infants born to mothers with TB).

Literature describing this early work often notes that the original culture of BCG bacteria was never saved, i.e., no bacteriologically identical samples were made. Instead, the original strain was distributed to several different laboratories around the world, where it was maintained under different conditions, thereby leading to the generation of bacteriologically distinct strains. As a result, vaccines currently marketed as BCG actually comprise a group of related vaccines with differing characteristics, e.g., potency. This is one of several issues complicating the interpretation of clinical trials in which BCG was evaluated for efficacy (see below).

One freeze-dried strain of BCG containing live bacteria (referred to as Tice) is currently manufactured and sold in the United States, with Food and Drug Administration approval for use in the prevention of TB (and recently also in the treatment of bladder cancer) (10). The Tice strain is administered by multiple puncture only, not by the intradermal method generally preferred for BCG vaccination.

It is generally believed that BCG does not prevent initial infection with tubercle bacilli. Instead, BCG enhances the cellular immune response to *M.tb.* (by mechanisms that are not fully understood), thereby lowering the risk of developing active disease. It also seems to reduce multiplication of bacilli and dissemination of the disease to various parts of the body, thereby lowering the risk of extrapulmonary TB (305). How HIV-related immunodeficiency affects BCG's initial or subsequent immunologic actions is not clear. However, because a functional T-cell im-

[1] *Mycobacterium bovis* can cause TB in humans who have extensive contact with infected animals or who drink milk laden with tubercle bacilli.

Figure 4-1—Summary of Estimates of the Efficacy of BCG Vaccines Against Tuberculosis

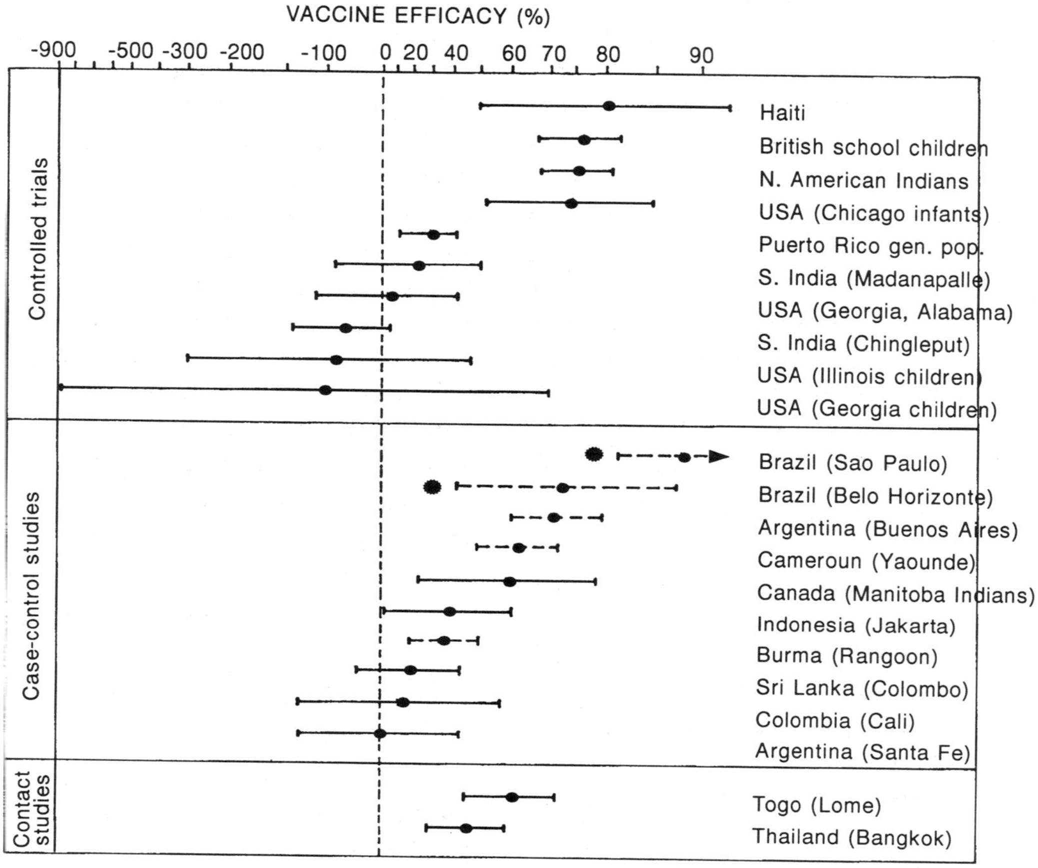

SOURCE: Reprinted with permission from P.E.M. Fine, "The BCG Story: Lessons From the Past and Implications for the Future," *Review of Infectious Diseases* 11(Suppl. 2):S353-S359, 1989.

mune system is believed necessary for BCG to work, it is not known whether the vaccine would protect against TB in HIV-infected individuals (103).

Unfortunately, there is currently no reliable immunologic measure of protective immunity to TB following BCG administration, so it is difficult to monitor and evaluate its effects. Tuberculin sensitivity (by skin testing) following BCG (referred to as a BCG-induced DHT response) does not correlate with protective immunity to TB (98).

Efficacy and Safety of BCG Vaccination

Ten major randomized clinical trials and many nonrandomized studies of BCG vaccination have been conducted in various populations since the 1930s (summarized in figure 4-1). These trials are noteworthy not only for their size (only the Salk polio vaccine trials involved more subjects), but also for the duration of followup. The most recent trial, begun in 1968, involved 115,000 subjects followed for 7.5 years in Chingleput, South India (327).

Despite the enormous international effort to determine the protective efficacy of BCG (defined as the percent reduction in risk of TB among BCG recipients, compared with similarly exposed nonvaccinated subjects), the issue remains unresolved; a strikingly broad range of protective efficacy, from zero (or negative) to 80 percent, was found (98,99). As a result, there are major differences in expert opinion on the subject, and a continuing controversy surrounding the analysis of the data (59,98).

Why the vaccine worked well in some study populations and failed in others is still not known and may never be known. Various biological and statistical factors accounting for the variability have been proposed and debated, including:

- variations among the strains of BCG used in the studies;
- confounding immunologic effects of widespread infection with other types of mycobacteria commonly found in soil and tap water in some areas, some of which can induce a similar immunologic effect against tubercle bacilli as BCG;
- regional differences in virulence of the tubercle bacilli;
- nutritional and genetic differences in the populations studied; and
- methodologic differences in trial design (59, 98,99).

Some or all of these factors, or others not yet identified, may have influenced the trial results, producing observed differences in efficacy. Current efforts to conduct a meta-analysis of the data may clarify some of these issues (198). Development of a reliable animal model to compare potencies of the BCG strains currently available may be necessary to select vaccines likely to be potent in the human population and to avoid those likely to be affected (63).

The data from these studies suggest that BCG offers greater protection for children against disseminated forms of TB (including a reduction in incidence of TB meningitis and miliary TB that ranges from 52 to 100 percent) than it offers against pulmonary TB (58,134,343).

Side effects and adverse reactions to BCG vaccination are rare in immunocompetent individuals (179,343). The increasing prevalence of HIV in some populations, however, has raised concern over the safety of BCG vaccination in immunodeficient individuals since BCG is an attenuated live vaccine and thereby poses potential risks of dissemination in immunodeficient individuals (42,238). Case reports of serious complications of BCG vaccination in HIV-infected infants (141,210) and adults with AIDS (11,33,341) have been reported. CDC notes that HIV-infected individuals may be at greater risk for complications from BCG vaccine, but current data are insufficient to determine the magnitude of the risk and level of immunodeficiency at which the effect might manifest (343).

Impact of BCG Vaccination on the Incidence of TB

Although BCG vaccination has long been conducted in many parts of the world with the intent of reducing the incidence of pulmonary TB in the population, its impact on the control of pulmonary TB is not easily discernible. The large burden of TB in many countries over the years suggests that even if BCG vaccination has reduced the incidence of TB (which some argue it must have, given the billions of doses administered over the years and some potential for benefit) (99), it is obviously not a sufficient strategy to prevent the disease. The degree to which it contributed to previous declines in TB incidence (e.g., in Western Europe) may never be known, given other contemporaneous factors, such as socioeconomic improvements and increased availability of anti-TB drugs. Within the next decade, the rising prevalence of HIV may substantially reduce the impact of BCG vaccination.

Most experts agree, however, that BCG may reduce the incidence of the serious (and noncontagious) childhood forms of TB (TB meningitis and other disseminated forms of TB). In some high-risk countries, BCG vaccination may provide good protection against these forms of the disease, but it is not likely to prevent transmission of pulmonary TB among young and older adults, who are the main sources of infection to children and other adults in the population. Ironically, global BCG vaccination campaigns may have actually contributed more to complacency about TB over the years, with a corresponding decline in interest in developing better methods of prevention and treatment, than to TB eradication itself (98).

BCG Vaccination Policy in the United States

BCG vaccination of children or adults has never been carried out on a routine basis in the United States. CDC cites two main reasons for this policy—a low risk of tuberculous infection in the general population, and the variable efficacy of the vaccine (378). In its most recent policy summary, however, CDC does recommend selected use of the vaccine in certain high-risk infants and children such as those with negative tuberculin skin tests who are in unavoidable and close contact with infectious individuals and who cannot be treated with INH preventive therapy, or those who are continuously exposed to individuals with MDR-TB. CDC also recommends BCG vaccination in:

> "...tuberculin-negative infants and children in groups in which the rate of new infections exceeds 1 percent per year and for whom the usual treatment and control programs are not effective. These groups include persons without regular access to health care, those for whom health care is culturally or socially unacceptable, and groups who have demonstrated an inability to use existing health care" (378).

It is not clear whether the rationale for this recommendation is narrow (i.e., to prevent the childhood disseminated forms of TB), or broad (i.e., to offer a prevention, albeit uncertain for those who are either unreachable or not covered by current TB control efforts). Previous policy statements issued by CDC and the American Thoracic Society made similar recommendations (6), although they were not limited to infants and children, also specifying "alcoholics, drug addicts, migrants, and refugees" as those without regular access to health care for whom BCG might be appropriate (170).

BCG vaccination may itself cause subsequent reaction to tuberculin skin tests, thereby making interpretation of the skin test more difficult in some cases. Currently, no reliable method for distinguishing between tuberculin skin test reactions caused by BCG and those caused by tuberculous infection exists (378) but the reaction due to BCG is believed to wane after 3 to 5 years (307). In general, some judgments can be made on the basis of the size of the tuberculin reaction (with "significant" reactions more likely indicating true infection), the individual's risk of infection, presence of BCG "scar," and how long ago BCG was given (291,378). Framed as a policy choice between alternative strategies for TB prevention, skin testing and preventive treatment have long been favored in the United State over mass BCG vaccination, even though efforts to deliver preventive treatment have not been widely implemented.

In its 1988 statement on BCG, CDC reversed its 1979 recommendation for high-risk HCWs to receive BCG vaccination, citing a lack of evidence for increased rates of infection or tuberculin skin test conversion among HCWs (343). They opted instead for promoting greater use of skin testing and preventive therapy and of hospital infection control measures.

Because of possible risks of adverse effects from BCG vaccination among individuals with HIV, CDC did not recommend BCG vaccination for anyone known or suspected to be infected with HIV, except in selected populations where the risk of TB is high (343). Further data on complications of BCG in HIV-infected individuals (most likely reported from developing countries) may help to clarify these issues for which there is little experience in the United States. Data on the efficacy of BCG in HIV-infected individuals are nonexistent. All previously mentioned clinical trials were conducted prior to 1980.

Issues Concerning Future Use of Vaccination Against TB

The current resurgence of TB in the United States highlights the continuing need for a vaccine that is effective and safe, particularly for individuals infected with HIV, who are at highest risk for developing active TB. Those who are tuberculin-negative and in close contact with individuals who have active, infectious MDR-TB, such as prison staff and inmates, HCWs and patients, and homeless shelter staff and residents, have the most to benefit from effective vaccination, along with HIV-seronegative individuals who are at high risk for becoming infected with HIV.

Until an improved vaccine is developed, an expanded role for BCG vaccination in HIV-seronegative (and ''asymptomatic'' HIV-seropositive) groups needs to be considered in light of the risks, possible benefits to the affected individuals, and potential drawbacks to infection monitoring and preventive treatment efforts.

The need for new, improved vaccines against TB was noted in CDC's recent ''National Action Plan to Combat MDR-TB.'' Ideally, such a vaccine would effectively prevent infection progressing to active TB and would not interfere with interpretation of tuberculin skin testing (166). In order to develop and test a new TB vaccine, a number of unresolved issues in TB immunology may need to be addressed, including: identification of immunogenic and virulence components of the tubercle bacillus and which of these elicit protective immune responses, characterization of these immune responses, and development of animal models for TB prevention that correlate well with human responses (363,373). The possibility of deriving an effective vaccine against TB using a genetically engineered recombinant BCG vaccine containing antigen-encoding genes has been explored in recent studies (3,313). NIAID is currently funding several research efforts aimed at developing a new TB vaccine (see chapter 7) (104).

Diagnosis and Treatment of Active TB 5

For tuberculosis (TB), as for many other infectious diseases, rapid and accurate diagnosis coupled with delivery of effective treatment are the central elements of medical and public health efforts to control the disease. Recent shifts in the nature of TB—notably, the increasing numbers of multidrug-resistant TB (MDR-TB) cases and the particular vulnerability to TB of individuals infected with the human immunodeficiency virus (HIV)—have heightened the need for improved methods of diagnosis and for shorter, simpler treatment regimens.

Diagnostic methods currently in use in many countries have remained unchanged for decades; the need for improved methods is acute, particularly in areas with a high prevalence of HIV. In the United States, newer diagnostic methods have been adopted in the past few years, but additional developments are needed to respond adequately to the recent rise in TB and MDR-TB. Deficiencies in the current diagnostic technology could seriously hamper efforts to control the spread of TB among HIV-infected populations in particular.

This chapter examines current needs and capabilities for diagnosis of active, infectious TB, along with the rationale and design of corresponding treatment regimens. The focus is primarily on pulmonary TB, rather than the various forms of extrapulmonary TB (TB in organs or tissues of the body other than the lung), because pulmonary TB is the predominant form and is the one responsible for transmission of the disease (see chapter 2). Details concerning the diagnosis and treatment of extrapulmonary TB can be found in several recent reviews (75,217,227). Treatment of noncontagious tuberculous infection, as distinct from active TB, and issues concerning skin testing for infection are discussed in chapter 4.

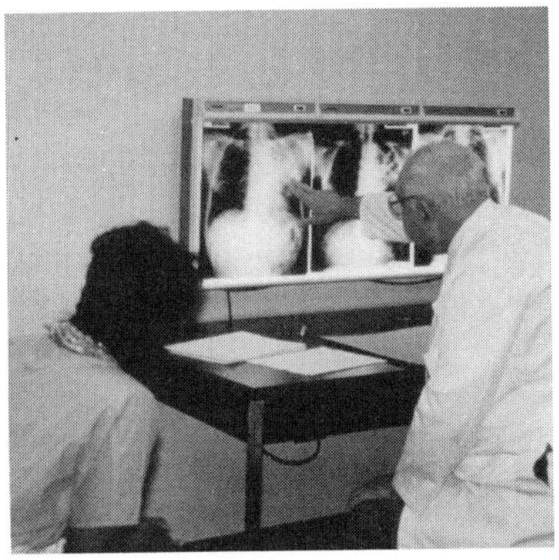

DIAGNOSIS OF TB AND RESISTANCE TO ANTI-TB DRUGS

Rapid, accurate diagnosis of TB allows for appropriate treatment to be initiated so that patients can be rendered noninfectious, cured of the disease, and prevented from relapsing at a later date. By causing delays in initiating appropriate treatment, diagnostic delays and errors can lead to the avoidable continuation and spread of TB. In many ways, current problems in diagnosis are no different from those of the past. It has long been recognized that the available methods are far from ideal, but their widespread acceptance suggests that they are adequate in most uncomplicated cases. Increasingly, however, the inadequacies of the current methods have become magnified in the face of rising drug-resistance and the need to prevent rapid spread of the disease among patients in congregate settings and among HIV-infected populations. Patients with HIV who develop active TB may be at increased risk for rapid death from TB if effective treatment is not begun promptly (14,174).

At present, there is no single, definitive, quick test for active TB. By necessity, diagnosis is based on a combination of clinical acumen (aided by an assessment of the patient's risk for TB, medical history, and clinical signs) and laboratory and x-ray findings (70). Clinical symptoms of active TB include a persistent cough, hemoptysis (coughing up of blood), weight loss, fatigue, night sweats, and fever (8).

The tuberculin skin test is the standard method for screening asymptomatic individuals for tuberculous infection (and possibly disease) (see chapter 4). However, because of a high rate of false negative reactions (and some false positives) in both immunocompetent and immunocompromised individuals with TB, the skin test is considered inadequate for diagnosing active disease (8).

The classic initial laboratory method for presumptively diagnosing active TB is the sputum smear. Samples of the patient's sputum (phlegm) are placed on a slide, stained with a dye for acid-fast bacilli (AFB), and examined under a light or fluorescent microscope (7,70). The sputum smear test is quick and inexpensive, but is useful only when positive; negative smears cannot be used to rule out TB. The smear test does not distinguish tubercle bacilli from other types of (nontuberculous) mycobacteria, nocardia, or some legionella and nor does it indicate the bacilli's susceptibility to anti-TB drugs. However, when considered with other indicators, the smear test is used to make a presumptive diagnosis (276). When the test shows AFB, it also allows an estimation of the number of bacilli present and being excreted, an indicator of the patient's degree of infectiousness (7).

The major limitation of the sputum smear is its inadequate sensitivity due in part to technician-variability: only 50 to 80 percent of patients with pulmonary TB may have positive sputum smears (276). The detection rate among patients with advanced stages of HIV-related immunosuppression may be even lower (70,174,236). Samples of other respiratory secretions, biopsy body fluids, gastrics washings, bone marrow aspirates, and urine sediments for staining and smear examination would be needed to rule out false negative results (8). In addition, false positives are an increasing problem, due to the high prevalence of nontuberculous mycobacterial infections in HIV-infected individuals.

Chest x-rays are also used to detect active TB. Typical findings of TB in immunocompetent adults include infiltrates in the upper lung areas and cavitation. In TB patients with HIV, chest x-ray findings are likely to be atypical (with more middle and lower lung lobe involvement, no cavitation, and hilar or mediastinal lymphadenopathy); in general, the more advanced the immunosuppression, the more atypical the radiographic signs of TB (215,236,242). Because of this and the likelihood of false negative sputum smears, diagnosis of TB in patients with HIV involves even more uncertainties than in immunocompetent patients.

Definitive diagnosis of TB has traditionally been based on specific identification of the causative organism, *Mycobacterium tuberculosis*, isolated from sputum, body fluids, or tissue and cultured in the laboratory (8). Positive culture examination is considered to be far more sensitive and specific than sputum smears, but is also more expensive and time-consuming (123,276). Typically, conventional culture tests require 3 to 6 weeks to generate results because of the organism's slow growth rate. Culture methods provide confirmation of suspected TB cases, but, by necessity, empiric treatment is usually begun before such results are available.

Diagnosis of active TB in children poses additional difficulties, since sputum smear and culture tests often do not reveal the presence of tubercle bacilli (which may be present, though in smaller numbers than in an adult). It is also difficult to distinguish tuberculous infection from active TB in children. Various indirect means are usually used to establish a presumptive diagnosis of TB in a child, including epidemiologic information about the child's exposure to an adult with active TB, tuberculin skin test results, chest x-ray findings, and physical examination for symptoms consistent with TB even though the child may be asymptomatic (302). Confirmation of active TB through culture examination is often more difficult in children because of the difficulty in collecting sputum samples and because of the even lower sensitivity of alternative fluids (such as gastric washings) for bacteriologic confirmation of TB (306).

In recent years, many laboratories responsible for processing TB specimens have incorporated more efficient methods for culture examination. An automated, radiometric method (known by its trade name BACTEC™), which detects growth of *M. tuberculosis* in a selective medium containing radiometric palmitic acid by measuring radioactive carbon dioxide given off by the bacteria, reduces the testing time to about 10 days (384). Gene probes specific for *M. tuberculosis* can also be used in conjunction with radiometric testing to shorten the time needed to identify tubercle bacilli. Another method, also producing faster definitive results, is based on detecting microcolonies of the organism grown on solid media and identifying them as *M. tuberculosis* by morphology (384).

Conventional methods for testing tubercle bacilli's drug susceptibility, using solid media and indirect testing, typically take 8 to 12 weeks to identify bacilli resistant to anti-TB drugs. The newer radiometric techniques, along with direct testing, which are also used to test for susceptibility to the five first-line drugs, take up to 3 weeks (133). Conventional drug susceptibility testing methods, taking several weeks longer, are used to test for resistance to other drugs and to confirm results of the radiometric studies (382).

Jacobs and colleagues recently reported a new laboratory method for rapid determination of drug-susceptibility (158). The technique is based on a light-producing reaction catalyzed by the firefly enzyme luciferase to distinguish drug-resistant and drug-sensitive tubercle bacilli, and can generate results in 2.3 days. It has not yet been adapted for clinical use.

TB diagnosis based on deoxyribonucleic (DNA) methods has recently been reported. At present, the most fully developed of these methods is one based on DNA amplification using the polymerase chain reaction (which allows the use of uncultured clinical specimens) followed by gene probes for DNA sequences specific for *M. tuberculosis* (44,281). Results can reportedly be obtained in 48 hours (89), although the test is not yet available for routine clinical use. An alternative to the use of radioactive isotopes in this method was recently reported (322). Other approaches, such as those based on immunoassay, are in developmental stages (70,122,188).

Delayed diagnosis was considered to be one of the main factors contributing to several of the recent nosocomial outbreaks of MDR-TB (discussed in chapters 3 and 4). Patients with TB who remained infectious for prolonged periods transmitted the disease to other patients and health care workers (HCWs). There were several likely reasons for this, including HCWs' failure to suspect TB, unusual clinical features of TB in these patient populations, and the lengthy period of time required for laboratory identification, confirmation, and reporting of drug-susceptibility results (174). In addition, adequate infection control precautions were either not taken or not maintained, permitting infectious patients to remain in contact with patients and staff (see chapter 4). In congregate settings, such as hospitals, prisons, nursing homes, and other sites, there is a premium on rapid, accurate diagnosis to reduce the risk of active transmission.

The increasing prevalence of MDR-TB creates additional need for a rapid capability to identify the resistance pattern in each case so that the initial period of infectiousness can be shortened by administration of appropriate drugs for treatment. Recent Centers for Disease Control and Prevention (CDC) recommendations state that during the initial period when specific drug resistance information is not yet known, patients should generally be treated initially with four drugs (8,366). CDC lists patients more likely to have drug-resistant TB as those:

- from high-prevalence areas of the United States or foreign countries; and
- who have been in contact with other patients already infected with MDR-TB, have cavitary disease, or have been previously treated for TB (382).

In patients with drug-susceptible TB or who are TB resistant to a single drug, the four-drug regimen should render him or her noninfectious within a short period and offer the eventual possibility of cure. The regimen may be inadequate, however, in patients with resistance to three or more of the drugs. These MDR-TB patients could remain infectious for prolonged periods, posing a risk of transmitting the disease to other patients, family, and institutional staff. In New York City, where the incidence of MDR-TB is the highest in the country, the prevalence of resistance to both INH and RIF may be as high as 19 percent, according to a recent survey (107). Delays in obtaining drug-susceptibility data create additional need for hospitals to implement infection control precautions and isolation procedures to protect other patients and staff. Treatment of patients with MDR-TB must rely on the more toxic and expensive second-line drugs (discussed later) or newer drugs with *in vitro* activity against tubercle bacilli.

TREATMENT OF ACTIVE TB

Fifty years ago, before antibiotics were available for use in treating TB, treatment involved mainly improved nutrition, extended bed rest (often in TB sanatoria or other specialized institutions) and on some forms of surgical intervention to remove part of the lung (127). Mortality rates averaged around 50 to 60 percent 5 years after completion of treatment (200).

The introduction of antibiotic drug treatment in the late 1940s and combined-drug regimens in the 1950s dramatically changed the outcome of TB treatment. Rather than spending long periods of time in sanatoria or hospitals, patients could be treated on an outpatient basis with oral drugs that quickly rendered them noninfectious. Hospitalization could be limited to patients who needed diagnostic evaluation, developed complications, or could not care for themselves (1). Surgical intervention became unnecessary in most cases. Generally, patients could be treated at home and could return to outside activities soon after treatment was initiated (178). Although it was not the case for the initial single antibiotic (streptomycin) regimen, the multidrug regimens have reduced mortality from TB to about 4 percent (236).

Since the 1940s, the theory and practice of antibiotic treatment for TB has undergone substantial change and refinement both in the combination of drugs used and in the overall duration of treatment. Streptomycin (SM) was the first antibiotic applied to TB, followed by isoniazid (INH), p-aminosalicylic acid (PAS), and ethambutol (EMB). The potential for effective treatment and cure of TB was quickly apparent, but the long duration of treatment required for cure (e.g., 18 to 24 months) suggested the need for better drugs. The subsequent availability and use in the 1960s and 1970s of two other drugs—rifampin (RIF) and lower doses of pyrazinamide (PZA)—permitted shorter regimens to be used.

During the past 20 years, no new drugs have replaced or supplemented the five main first-line drugs—INH, RIF, PZA, EMB, and SM. Numerous other drugs of lesser effectiveness and greater toxicity have also been available as second-line drugs. During this time, clinical research and practice have focused on determining the optimal use of the first-line drugs. These efforts have resulted in revised combinations and durations of treatment for enhancing effectiveness, reducing toxicity, improving compliance, and reducing costs. Current regimens call for more intensive use of these drugs over shorter periods of time—now 6 months, compared with the previous 18- to 24-month schedule of treatment. The 6-month period appears to be the irreducible minimum for the currently available drugs; further reductions in treatment time will depend on the development of new agents.

Clinical trials conducted internationally by the British Medical Research Council (BMRC) and the U.S. Public Health Service produced the evidence for these changes in practice. The first East African/BMRC study reported in 1977 demonstrated that treatment could be shortened from 18 to 9 months by using RIF along with INH and SM, while still producing cures in over 95 percent of patients (86). Subsequent BMRC studies conducted in Hong Kong, Africa, and Singapore helped to define alternative drug combinations, minimum durations of therapy, and frequency of drug administration. As of the early 1980s, these trials showed that a regimen of PZA added to the first 2 months of daily INH, RIF, and SM therapy could elicit cures in 99 percent of patients, that 6 months was the minimum period of time necessary for such cure rates, and that intermittent therapy could be used without reducing effectiveness (154).

A recently reported randomized, multicenter study conducted by CDC demonstrated the effectiveness of shorter combination regimens in U.S. patients with TB (62). The study compared the effectiveness and toxicity of a 6-month regimen with the "standard" 9-months regimen among 1,451 newly diagnosed adults patients with pulmonary TB. The study did not include immunocompromised patients such as those with metastatic cancer or with HIV. Patients receiving the 6-month regimen were further randomized to treatment consisting of individual antibiotics taken together and treatment with Rifater™, a single, combination capsule containing the same three antibiotics. The 9-month regimen consisted of INH and RIF given daily for 36 weeks; the 6-month regimen consisted of the same two drugs given daily for 24 weeks, plus a third drug, PZA, given daily for the first 8 weeks of therapy. Patients randomized to the Rifater™ regimen received all three drugs for the first 2 months, followed by INH and RIF (Rifamate™ combination tablets) during the remaining 4 months.

The study found the 6-month regimen of the three drugs produced better results than the standard two-drug, 9-month regimen. Among patients on the 6-month regimen, about 95 percent had negative sputum cultures by 16 weeks of therapy (compared with 90 percent of patients on the 9-month regimen). Patients taking Rifater™ had even higher conversion rates than patients on the original 6-month regimen. The two groups had similar rates of relapse (about 3 percent) by 96 weeks after treatment and similar rates of adverse drug reactions (about 7 percent), although the 6-month regimen was associated with a higher rate of nonhepatotoxic reactions (primarily gastrointestinal upset and joint pain). The efficacy of both regimens was very high—over 96 percent of the patients were cured. An important practical benefit to the shorter regimen

AMERICAN LUNG ASSOCIATION

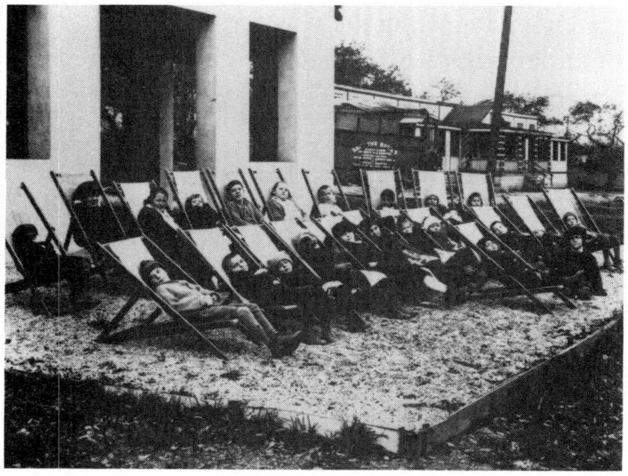

During the 1920s, before the discovery of drugs to treat tuberculosis, sanatoriums and other TB hospitals were the centerpiece of treatment that focused on keeping the patient hearty. Sanatoriums were phased out during the 1950s and 1960s.

was that a higher proportion of patients successfully completed therapy.

Rationale for Antimicrobial Treatment of TB

Theoretically, the ultimate goal of treatment is to rid the body of tubercle bacilli before irreversible physiologic damage occurs in the lung, but in practice, the specific goals are to render the patient noninfectious, prevent the emergence of drug-resistant disease, and to allow cure without subsequent relapse. Certain characteristics of tubercle bacilli and their sites of infection in the body are important in determining how this can be accomplished. In general, tubercle bacilli replicate slowly and can remain dormant in the body for many years. Under favorable physiologic conditions for bacilli, they double in number every 20 hours, but in unfavorable conditions, they divide much less frequently or remain dormant for prolonged periods. This characteristic accounts for the long periods of treatment necessary to eradicate all dividing bacilli in the body and for occasional relapses despite apparently effective treatment.

Current anti-TB drugs kill tubercle bacilli only during periods of replication and activity. Conditions are most favorable for the bacilli's active metabolism in the open cavities of the lung, where the largest bacterial population is likely to be in an adult with pulmonary TB. In immunocompetent hosts, bacilli in closed caseous lesions and in macrophages are relatively slow metabolizers and replicate only intermittently.

A theoretical model for characterizing different subpopulations of tubercle bacilli in the body and for explaining the differential action of the major antibacterial drugs has been proposed (192). These four subpopulations are distinguished according to growth rates and sites of infection in the body.

One group is the subpopulation of bacilli responsible for the infectiousness of TB. It is characterized by active metabolism, relatively rapid growth rates, and large numbers of bacilli, including drug-resistant ones. These bacilli are usually found in the wall of lung cavitary lesions, where conditions favorable for growth occur (high oxygen and low acidity), and in the sputum. Bacilli are also found in the sputum. They are particularly vulnerable to the bactericidal action of INH, which kills rapidly growing bacilli during the first few days of treatment.

A second group of tubercle bacilli is characterized by slower or intermittent growth in acidic environments within cells (and possibly also outside of cells where there is an inflammatory response). There are probably fewer of these types of bacilli in the body, but they may persist despite short-term bactericidal treatment. They can also cause subsequent relapses later. PZA is believed to be most active in killing these bacilli.

A third group is believed to persist within cells and either remain dormant for long periods or undergo intermittent activity. These are thought to be treated most effectively with RIF. A fourth population of bacilli may be largely dormant, not affected by any of the antibiotic drugs, existing within solid caseous lesions and probably inaccessible to host immune forces (216).

Tubercle bacilli can undergo mutation in genes that confers resistance to the effects of anti-TB drugs. It is estimated that 1 in 100,000 to 1 in 100 million bacilli are initially resistant to any single drug used against TB. These few bacilli can, under certain conditions such as treatment with only one drug or erratic drug taking, become the predominant cell type in a bacterial population, creating single- or multidrug-resistant TB. Treatment with an adequate combination of drugs can prevent the emergence of a population dominated by drug-resistant bacilli (75).

Current Treatment Regimens

Combinations of antibiotic drugs with overlapping functions are used in current treatment regimens to attack the various distinct groups of tubercle bacilli in the body (75). Anti-TB drugs are generally classified as bactericidal (producing rapid killing of bacilli) or sterilizing (killing the last surviving, slowly metabolizing bacilli over the long term). The major bactericidal drug is INH, which is capable of producing a rapid decrease in the number of living bacilli in the sputum at the beginning of treatment and rapidly reducing the bacillary load in the patient. RIF and PZA are the most potent sterilizing drugs. Their use allowed the overall duration of treatment to be reduced to 6 months while minimizing relapse rates after initially successful therapy (110,192). INH and RIF (and to a lesser extent EMB and SM) are considered the most effective drugs in preventing the emergence of drug-resistant bacilli.

Corresponding to the different roles of these drugs, current regimens consist of two phases of treatment: an initial intensive bactericidal phase intended to eliminate quickly the bulk of tubercle bacilli from most body sites, followed by a longer-term sterilizing phase intended to eliminate the remaining bacilli. The initial regimen involves the daily use of four drugs (INH, RIF, PZA and EMB or SM). The total duration of treatment is 6 months, although several variations of this regimen (in terms of types of drugs and frequency of administration) are also used (366). In general, the various combinations of the four-drug regimens yield cure rates of 98 percent or more and relapse rates of less than 3 percent (8).

These drugs are not without side effects, the most serious of which is hepatitis (inflammation of the liver) (380). Usually associated with INH, but also with RIF and PZA, drug-related hepatitis is more frequent among older patients, those with preexisting liver disease, and those who abuse alcohol (these are also risk factors for hepatitis unrelated to INH, PZA, and RIF) (114). Other common adverse reactions include: hypersensitivity reactions, along with gastrointestinal distress (caused by RIF), hyperuricemia (caused by PZA), vertigo or hearing loss and nephrotoxicity (caused by SM), and optic neuritis (caused by EMB). However, the more serious and more frequent adverse effects are generally associated with use of the second-line drugs (178).

The patient's improvement with treatment is measured first by clinical improvement such as loss of fever, reduction in coughing, increased appetite, and weight gain. Reduction in numbers of tubercle bacilli in the patient's sputum also indicates improvement. Failure of sputum culture conversion or reappearance of viable bacilli in the sputum following initial clearing may signal treatment failure. Subsequent signs of treatment failure include a worsening of clinical status and progression of disease as detected on chest radiography. Patients are usually monitored on a monthly basis for adverse effects and treatment response (178). Within 2 to 3 months of treatment, about 90 percent of patients with uncomplicated, pulmonary TB would have negative sputum cultures. Patients with drug-resistant TB may show persistently positive sputum cultures. The treatment of TB in children follows the same principles as in adults, although diagnosing and monitoring progress with treatment is more complex and necessitates the use of various indirect indices (303).

Treatment of TB in Individuals with AIDS

Current recommendations for treatment of TB in patients with AIDS specify the same combination of antibiotics as for immunocompetent TB patients (344,366,378).

In general, TB is treatable in individuals with HIV. Although experience is limited, reports to date suggest that HIV-infected patients, even those with advanced stages of immunodeficiency, can undergo rapid elimination of tubercle bacilli from the sputum, clinical improvement, and low rates of relapse following standard anti-TB treatment (232,290,321). Most documented cases of treatment failure in patients with HIV have been linked to incomplete treatment or poor absorption of anti-TB drugs (117,290).

Nevertheless, several added complexities in treating TB in patients with HIV exist. Coexisting infections and other AIDS-associated disorders require treatments that may interact with the antibiotics used to treat TB. High rates of toxicities and drug reactions, especially to RIF, have been noted in TB patients with AIDS (103,212,290). Many of the adverse reactions were considered serious enough to drop RIF from the regimen, making a cure of TB in these cases much more difficult. For a variety of reasons, toxicities from anti-TB drugs may be more difficult to interpret in patients with AIDS and TB (230).

Another complicating factor is that various types of disseminated or extrapulmonary TB appear to be more common among patients with HIV (100,230). Some of these (particularly central nervous system TB) may pose more immediate risks and are more difficult to diagnose and treat (212).

Completion of treatment, a critical factor in treatment of all TB patients, may be even more critical to successful outcomes in patients with HIV. At the same time, some subgroups of patients such as intravenous drug users with HIV may be at higher risk for treatment failure. Chapter 6 examines this issue in greater detail.

Finally, although patients with AIDS usually respond to TB therapy, the optimal duration of therapy to prevent relapse following treatment in these patients is uncertain (212,230). Initial recommendations for longer courses of treatment were based on case reports of several patients found to have progressive disease despite adequate treatment (319) and on prior difficulties with the treatment of other opportunistic infections. Recent reports of successful outcomes with 6-month regimens (290,321) cast doubt on the necessity of prolonged treatment, but clinical trials with long-term followup will be needed to determine the efficacy of short-course treatment in larger groups of HIV patients. In the meantime, HIV-infected patients treated for TB probably need frequent followup, including regular mycobacterial examinations, for life (230).

Treatment of Multidrug-Resistant TB

When SM was introduced in the late 1940s as the first chemotherapeutic agent against TB, it was administered singly. The first group of patients treated with SM responded well initially, but in a short time, relapsed with large numbers of SM-resistant tubercle bacilli. SM had effectively killed the susceptible bacilli but not the resistant ones, which had been present in small numbers from the outset by random mutation.

It was soon recognized that the use of a single antimicrobial drug in treating TB would lead predictably to the development of resistant disease, and that multiple drugs to which the bacilli were susceptible would be necessary to prevent the development of drug resistance. The use of combination chemotherapy to treat TB has been standard practice since the early 1950s, initially with INH, SM, and PAS, next with INH, SM, and EMB, then INH and RIF, and now with four drugs until a patient's drug susceptibility test results are known (287,366,382).

Given the current prevalence of MDR-TB in the United States, such a four-drug regimen is estimated to be adequate for over 95 percent of

TB patients (25). The remaining 4 to 5 percent are resistant to 2 or more drugs in the current recommended regimens. Cases of resistance of up to seven drugs have been documented in recent outbreaks of MDR-TB in several New York City hospitals and prisons (382). In addition, patients with bacilli resistant to as many as 11 drugs have recently been reported (118).

Failure to complete a full course of appropriate treatment is a major cause of MDR-TB. Patients on combination-drug therapy who stop taking all medications at the same time may ultimately relapse, but with bacilli showing the same-drug susceptibility pattern as before. The recurrent disease in such cases would be treatable with the same combination of drugs. In contrast, patients who take their medications erratically or who stop taking only one or two of the drugs while continuing the others may relapse with TB resistant to one or several of the medications (267). In these cases, treatment of recurrent disease requires a different combination of drugs. The success of further treatment depends, in part, on the effectiveness of the remaining drugs that can be used. Patients who remain inadequately treated may also be capable of transmitting MDR-TB to others.

Data derived from a number of clinical trials conducted overseas by the BMRC suggest that patients with bacilli resistant to either INH or SM can be treated effectively with regimens initially containing four drugs (resulting in 94 to 97 percent cure rates in 6-month regimens), since the other 3 drugs would be usable (194). Resistance to RIF, however, poses a greater risk of treatment failure (194). Successful outcome of treatment is even less likely if there is resistance to both INH and RIF, the two most active anti-TB drugs currently available. High treatment failure rates and overall mortality among HIV-infected individuals with MDR-TB have recently been reported (100,118).

Drug regimens for MDR-TB are determined on a case-by-case basis, beginning with information derived from the patient's medical history (e.g., prior drugs taken for TB) and drug-susceptibility testing. Cases resistant to two or more of the first-line drugs would be treated with a combination of remaining first-line drugs, second-line drugs (capreomycin, kanamycin, ethionamide, cycloserine, and p-aminosalicylic acid and amikacin), often for 18 to 24 months or longer after conversion of sputum cultures.

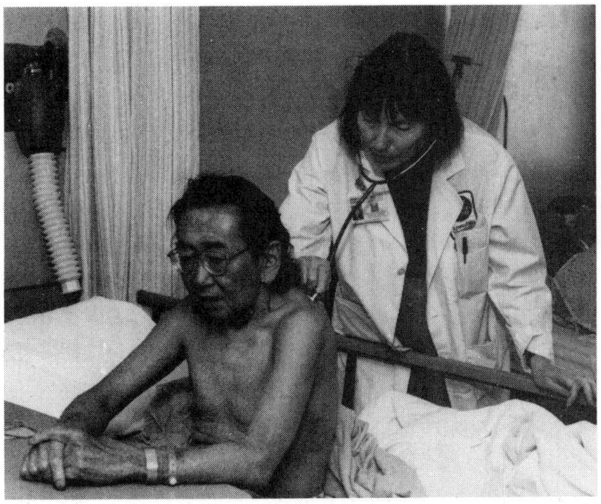

AMERICAN LUNG ASSOCIATION

Individuals with active, drug-susceptible TB, like this one at Bellevue Hospital in New York City, are often hospitalized during the initial period of their treatment while they are still infectious. Patients with drug-resistant TB may require longer hospitalizations.

A number of other drugs have been less extensively studied for anti-TB activity, and are not yet approved (because of insufficient data on efficacy) for the treatment of TB—clofazimine, quinolones (sparfloxacin and ofloxacin) (153). Reliable data to judge the effectiveness of these second-line drugs are lacking, but anecdotal experience suggests that they are much less effective and much more likely to lead to serious toxic effects (287). Adjunctive surgery to remove tissue (usually in the lung) heavily infected with tubercle bacilli is sometimes used as a treatment of last resort in patients with localized lung disease for whom drug treatment is inadequate (116). In general, treatment of MDR-TB requires more complex interventions, longer hospitalization and more extensive laboratory monitoring.

Beginning in 1990, widespread shortages of certain anti-TB drugs occurred in the United States (224,352). A number of contributing factors have been identified, including various problems within the generic drug industry, the reliance on sole suppliers of a bulk drug (often outside the United States), single U.S. manufacturers of the finished drug product, a low demand for anti-TB drugs overall, and low profit margins for drug companies manufacturing these drugs (189). In April 1992, CDC began to make PAS and SM available through an investigational new drug agreement with the Food and Drug Administration (FDA). FDA has worked with U.S. manufacturers to reestablish production and supplies of the affected drugs. As discussed in chapter 7, the FDA has also begun offering a variety of incentives to pharmaceutical companies to develop new anti-TB drugs, such as granting orphan drug status, conducting expedited review of applications, offering accelerated approval with the development of surrogate markers (interim outcomes), and accepting foreign clinical data (225).

New Approaches to Treatment

The rising prevalence of MDR-TB and the complexities of treating TB in patients with HIV have heightened the need for new anti-TB drugs, shorter regimens, and better methods of drug delivery.

Combination tablets containing three of the first-line drugs such as Rifater™, containing INH, RIF, and PZA, have been developed (192), but are not commercially available in the United States. In 1993, a new drug application to permit marketing of Rifater™ in the United States was submitted to the FDA (119). Rifamate™, a combination tablet containing INH and RIF, is FDA-approved and available; 40 percent of RIF prescribed in the United States is currently given as Rifamate™ (119). Some data are available on the effectiveness of combination preparations compared with the use of the same drugs given separately. In two BMRC studies, conflicting results were obtained in clinical trials, but in the recent study reported by Combs and colleagues, Rifater™ was found to be effective, although it was associated with a higher rate of adverse effects (62). Incorporation of these combined preparations into TB treatment, however, could possibly increase the overall success rate and help prevent the development of MDR-TB resulting from erratic drug taking or inadequate prescribing. One disadvantage of the combined preparations is that the regimen cannot be selectively modified to reduce adverse effects of component drugs without switching to individual drugs or discontinuing therapy altogether.

Intermittent therapy of equivalent effectiveness (twice or thrice weekly instead of daily administration) in the sterilizing phase of treatment improves chances for supervision of outpatient therapy, for reducing overall costs of treatment, and lowering drug toxicities (61). Further experimentation with even less frequent administration may depend on the use of drugs with longer duration of effect in the body (such as rifamycins). In this context, rifamycins are currently being studied in clinical trials in China (192). An optimal anti-TB agent would be bactericidal for all populations of bacilli within a very short period of time, orally administered or injectable in a single dose, and free of toxicities. Other drugs being investigated for this purpose include fluoroquinolones, rifamycin derivatives, and phenazines (127).

Alternative methods of drug delivery have been discussed but are not yet ready for clinical evaluation. Some of these include implantable devices containing drugs for slow release into the bloodstream (similar in design to the Norplant™ device for contraception), and the use of liposomes as carriers for drugs directly to specific sites in the body. Immunotherapeutic approaches are also under investigation.

Table 5-1—Trends in Drug Costs for Treating Tuberculosis in a 165 lb (75 kg) Patient, 1986-92: An Uncomplicated Case Versus a Case Resistant to INH and RIF[a]

Uncomplicated case:

Drug	Daily dose	Duration	1986 cost	1990 cost	1992 cost
Isonizaid	300 mg	180 days	$ 5.04	$ 6.50	$ 8.50
Rifampin	600 mg	180 days	106.20	159.30	165.30
Pyrazinamide	25 mg/kg	60 days	98.00	160.00	179.20
			$209.24	**$325.80**	**$353.00**

Average annual percentage increase in cost, 1986-92: 9.1%

A case resistant to INH and RIF:

Drug	Daily dose	Duration	1986 cost	1990 cost	1992 cost
Pyrazinamide	25 mg/kg	540 days	$ 882.00	$1,440.00	$1,613.00
Ethambutol	15 mg/kg	540 days	690.00	1,246.00	1,610.00
Streptomycin	15 mg/kg	120 days	138.00	192.00	206.00
Ethionamide	20 mg/kg	540 days	890.00	1,458.00	1,691.00
Ciprofloxacin	1500 mg	540 days	NA	3,000.00	3,600.00
			$2,600.00	**$7,338.00**	**$8720.00***

Average annual percentage increase in cost, 1986-92 (without Ciprofloxacin): 12.0%

*Add ofloxacin=$4,080.00
Add amikacin=$27,648.00
Add clofazimine=$71.00

KEY: NA = not available; mg = milligram; kg = kilogram (of patient body weight).

[a] Treatment costs based on median prices given in table 5-2. Costs are for an entire recommended treatment cycle. Estimates include drug costs only.

SOURCE: U.S. Department of Health and Human Services, Public Health Service, Centers for Disease Control and Prevention, Division of Tuberculosis Elimination, 1993.

The Cost of Drugs for Tuberculosis Treatment

The purchase of anti-TB drugs varies by jurisdiction and can be done by State or local health departments, or by other organizations. The drugs' prices can vary depending on manufacturer, the quantities purchased, and other terms of the sale (190). In addition, not all States use all the same drugs or dose forms. In response to price concerns over anti-TB drugs, CDC recently completed a survey of 14 jurisdictions (13 States and Baltimore City) to gather data on the last prices they paid for their pharmaceuticals in 1986, 1990, and 1992. Tables 5-1 and 5-2 present CDC's results. Table 5-1 gives estimates prepared by CDC of the costs of two possible drug regimens for a 165-pound (75-kg) adult: one for uncomplicated TB, the other a TB case resistant to INH and RIF. Table 5-2 presents data on increases in individual dosage forms of most first-line and second-line anti-tuberculosis drugs.[1] Although prices paid by State and local health departments vary and the precise number of drugs required for treatment is different for each patient, these estimates still give a sense of the resources needed for drugs to treat a TB patient as well as

[1] Some dosage forms were purchased by only a small subset of States. According to CDC, its discussions with some State and local authorities revealed that part of the increase in prices is due to the growing unwillingness of manufacturers to enter into contracts with public health authorities to supply drugs over time at a set, discounted price. Some of the range in prices is also due to the fact that some municipalities purchase in bulk under contract, while others lack the volume to do so (190).

Table 5-2—Trends in Tuberculosis Drug Prices: Results of U.S. Centers for Disease Control and Prevention Survey

Drug	Drug form and package size	1992 number States ordering	1992 price range	1992 median price	1990 median price	1986 median price	Percent increase 1990-92
Isoniazid	100 mg 100/bottle	14	$ 1.00-3.00	$ 1.75	$ 1.25	$ .85	40%
Isoniazid	300 mg 30/bottle	13	1.07-2.71	1.41	1.09	.84	29
Isoniazid	300 mg 100/bottle	5	1.64-3.65	2.41	2.33	1.36	3
Isoniazid	Syrup 1 pint bottle	14	6.25-12.86	9.55	7.72	8.29	24
Rifampin and Isoniazid	Combo pack 30 day	11	27.36-31.89	31.40	27.36	19.60	15
Rifampin	150 mg 30/bottle	13	33.30-40.00	33.45	29.60	18.20	13
Rifampin	300 mg 60/bottle	14	26.10-59.04	27.25	26.55	17.70	3
Pyrazinamide	500 mg 100/bottle	6	65.49-75.12	71.70	60.97	38.42	18
Pyrazinamide	500 mg 500/bottle	9	280.00-359.28	326.63	292.63	188.62	12
Ethambutol	100 mg 100/bottle	10	19.73-30.25	29.18	24.05	16.37	21
Ethambutol	400 mg 100/bottle	7	97.66-103.75	101.57	78.87	53.82	29
Ethambutol	400 mg 1000/bottle	7	730.00-925.54	889.94	718.67	500.13	24
Streptomycin	1 gm vial	2	1.75-1.84	1.79	1.67	1.32	7
Streptomycin	2.5 gm vial	1	1.84	1.84	N/A	N/A	N/A
Streptomycin	5.0 gm vial	2	4.95-6.95	5.95	4.96	3.25	20
Paraamino salicyclicacid	500 mg 500/bottle	3	34.48-49.00	41.86	33.70	14.80	24
Ethionamide	250 mg 100/bottle	12	56.97-118.24	103.88	89.51	52.87	16
Capreomycin	1 gm 10 ml	9	16.25-21.07	18.80	14.84	11.95	27
Kanamycin	1 gm 3 ml	6	.75-22.60	.98	.75	1.40	31
Cycloserine	250 mg 40/bottle	10	89.99-115.50	108.85	86.10	34.78	26
Ciprofloxacin	250 mg 100/bottle	1	175.50	175.50	N/A	N/A	N/A
Ciprofloxacin	500 mg 100/bottle	8	108.13-236.85	225.27	94.12	75.00	133
Ciprofloxacin	750 mg 100/bottle	9	117.30-350.11	195.57	180.89	N/A	8
Clofazimine	50 mg 100/bottle	2	5.40-9.60	7.50	N/A	N/A	N/A
Clofazimine	100 mg 100/bottle	3	5.10-18.50	11.80	17.06	14.29	N/A
Ofloxacin	400 mg 50/bottle	4	15.88-154.15	136.25	N/A	N/A	N/A
Amikacin	1 gm	1	51.02	51.02	31.20	31.21	64
Pyridoxine	25 mg 100/bottle	2	.59-1.00	.80	N/A	N/A	N/A
Pyridoxine	50 mg 100/bottle	3	.84-1.70	.95	.85	.67	12

KEY: gm = gram; mg = milligram; N/A = not applicable.

SOURCE: Office of Technology Assessment, 1993, based on data from U.S. Department of Health and Human Services, Public Health Services, Centers for Disease Control and Prevention, 1993.

the upward trend in their prices (190). The costs of the regimen for uncomplicated TB described in table 5-1 rose an average over 9 percent per year between 1986 and 1992, a rate significantly higher than inflation during these years.

Delivery of Treatment for Tuberculosis 6

Despite the high potential for cure with current anti-TB treatment regimens, actual achievement of such cure in practice is far less certain. The multidrug and long-term nature of current treatment make the attainment of cure an exercise in perseverance. As described in chapter 5, treatment in uncomplicated cases typically involves taking 3 to 4 different drugs together on a daily, twice-weekly, or thrice-weekly schedule continuously for 6 months or more.[1]

Furthermore, some of the drugs cause unpleasant side effects or toxic reactions, so treatment also involves regular medical monitoring and substitution of different drugs, if necessary, in order to minimize adverse effects. Even though symptoms usually abate early in treatment and infectiousness may be quickly reduced, regular and complete administration of anti-TB drugs is necessary for eventual cure, prevention of relapse, and avoidance of drug-resistant disease. An adequate course of treatment for drug-sensitive TB is generally an arduous task, requiring a continual effort on the part of both patients and health care workers over a long, uninterrupted period of time.

In a broader sense, the achievement of cure with current treatment also depends on the quality and availability of local treatment services—complete case reporting, rapid and accurate diagnosis, appropriate prescription and provision of treatment, sustained followup of each case, and education of health professionals and patients concerning the disease and its treatment. Although efforts combining all of these activities are needed to control the spread of TB, methods of treatment

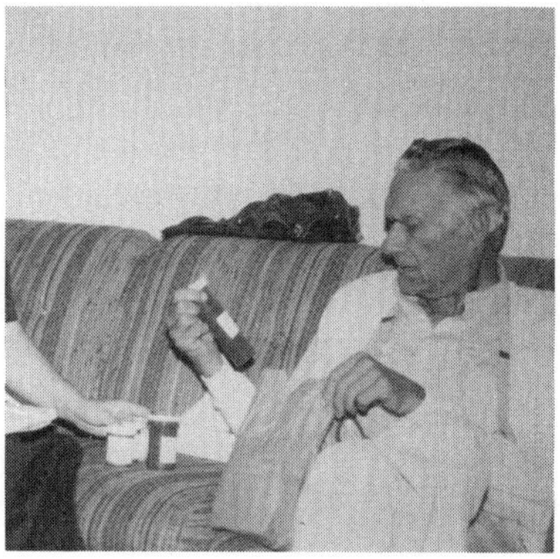

[1] In more complicated cases, such as those with resistance to two or more drugs, treatment involves taking at least 4 different drugs a day for 12 to 24 months, or even longer, in addition to more extensive medical care in a hospital or long-term care facility.

delivery and followup that foster close supervision and support of each patient are particularly important in the prevention and control of multidrug-resistant TB (MDR-TB).

Various social problems, such as homelessness, substance abuse, and poverty, increase the difficulty of assuring that patients receive regular and continuous treatment for TB in many areas of the United States. For some patients, access to other health services and social assistance, such as treatment for substance abuse, provision of stable housing, or mental health services, may play a critical role in their ability to make use of available TB treatment services and to adjust to a long-term treatment schedule (83).

Patients with active TB who do not receive an adequate course of treatment face the prospect of a progressively deteriorating condition and a substantial risk of dying from the disease within a short period of time. Moreover, for the patient's family, coworkers, and community, consequences of treatment failure include the risk of further spread of tuberculous infection to others, producing more cases of active TB and MDR-TB. Although drug-resistant tuberculous infection can be transmitted from person to person, virtually all strains of drug-resistant bacilli initially develop from erratic or inappropriate treatment in individuals with drug-susceptible TB. Furthermore, co-infection with the human immunodeficiency virus (HIV) shortens the time between tuberculous infection and active TB, further heightening the medical and public health significance of treatment failure.

Since the recent upturn in TB case rates, health officials have begun reexamining various strategies for improving the delivery of care for TB patients and for reducing the probability of treatment failure. Recent increases in MDR-TB cases, as in New York City (107), indicate that the inadequacy and ineffectiveness of current treatment delivery services are relevant issues for Federal and State policymakers to examine.

This chapter summarizes available data indicating the magnitude of the problem of treatment failure, and then briefly reviews the literature concerning factors involved in treatment failure. The final section summarizes various types of treatment delivery strategies that have been proposed to augment current services.

MAGNITUDE OF THE PROBLEM

Outcome data based on samples of U.S. TB case reports suggest that approximately 75 percent of U.S. patients being treated for TB complete treatment within a 12-month period and that 80 percent take their medication on a continuous basis (136). These aggregate data are derived from annual program management reports submitted on a voluntary basis to the Centers for Disease Control and Prevention (CDC) by some State and local TB programs, separately from the mandatory "Report of a Verified Case of Tuberculosis" (RVCT) surveillance system (see chapter 3). Beginning in 1993, the RVCT system will be expanded to include reporting of data on treatment completion and outcome in individual cases (363).

Before 1985, these data were reported as the percentage of patients completing 12 continuous months of treatment within a 24-month period. Since 1985, the reporting criteria have been changed (reflecting the use of shorter treatment regimens) to completion of 6 continuous months of treatment within a 12-month period. Before this change in reporting criteria the average percentage of patients completing treatment rose steadily from 69 percent in 1970 to 89 percent in 1985 (333a). At the same time, the sample size increased from 24 reporting areas in 1970 to 79 areas in 1985. Whether a real increase in the average completion rate during this period occurred is not known. Increased ascertainment of data could account for the change. Since 1985, the average rate of completion has changed little, varying between 74 and 78 percent, while the number of reporting areas increased from 82 to 93 (333a).

As of 1991, 93 reporting areas (including States, counties, and cities) were included in this database, corresponding to about three-quarters of all cases reported that year. No information is available from the remaining one-quarter of cases not reported in this system; to the extent that areas with poor reporting capabilities may also have deficiencies in other TB control services, the reported data may underestimate the average U.S. rate of treatment failure. Even if the data were complete, however, a single national average rate of treatment completion reveals only limited information about the nature of the problem, because of the wide variation in completion rates among programs and regions. For example, in the late 1980s, cities such as Chicago, New York, and the District of Columbia reported completion rates ranging from 54 to 60 percent, while Dallas, San Francisco, and El Paso reported rates above 94 percent. Outcome data for patients in Los Angeles were not reported at all, and are not reflected in the national average data (31). The specific reasons for these differences have not yet been determined. According to the National TB Action Plan, CDC plans to evaluate and compare TB control programs with the highest and lowest rates of treatment completion rates, in order to identify aspects of service delivery that contribute to successful outcomes of treatment (363).

Additional information about the extent of the problem in different populations or regions is available from various published reports on groups of patients undergoing treatment for TB. For example, in a multicenter clinical trial conducted by the Public Health Service (PHS) in 22 TB clinics around the country enrolling a total of 1,451 patients, only 61 percent of patients on a 6-month regimen and 51 percent of patients on a 9-month regimen completed their treatment for TB. Patients participating in this trial were treated under actual program conditions in effect in their local area; in general, treatment was self-administered (not directly supervised by program staff), although some incentives and educational interventions were offered (62).

In another paper, 80 TB patients treated between 1978 and 1982 in a hospital-based general outpatient clinic were compared with 104 patients treated between 1982 and 1987 in a hospital-based outpatient clinic specializing in TB treatment (385). The latter was designed specifically to improve followup of each case and maximize patients' abilities to stay on treatment.[2] In this setting, only 12 percent of patients completed treatment in the general outpatient clinic, whereas 86 percent of patients in the specialized clinic completed treatment.

The most widely cited report of treatment failure describes a group of 224 consecutive patients with TB admitted to Harlem Hospital in New York City during the first 9 months of 1988 (45). Of the 178 patients who were discharged while still on treatment, 89 percent were lost to followup service and did not complete their prescribed regimens. Forty-eight of these patients were later readmitted to the hospital with active TB; 40 were later discharged while still on treatment again; at least 35 of these patients were again lost to followup. Patients in this group who were homeless or alcoholic were significantly less likely than the other patients to complete treatment in the outpatient setting. Although the report states that patients discharged from the hospital were given an appointment for followup care at the hospital's chest clinic, no other details of their management at discharge or at that clinic were given.

At present, there are no national data on rates of cure, failure, or relapse among TB patients, since there has been no system for collecting and reporting such data to CDC. Some local programs may collect such data, but do not generally make the data available. Annual reports published by the New York City Department of Health and the

---

[2] For example, they used nurse specialists to follow each patients' progress, offering combination drug preparations, and provided money for public transportation to the clinic.

City of Chicago Department of Health, include detailed information on the epidemiology of TB in New York City and Chicago, respectively, but no data on outcome of treatment (56,57). As of 1993, CDC's expanded RCVT system will reportedly include such data.

FACTORS INVOLVED IN TREATMENT OUTCOME

The medical and public health literature contains ample recognition of the difficulty of achieving successful outcomes in patients with TB using available long-term treatment regimens. Some experts noted the problem as early as the 1950s when outpatient treatment using anti-TB drugs first became available (105,266). Analysis of the underlying causes appears uneven, however, with greater emphasis on patients' behavioral and social characteristics and much less on factors relating to the delivery of treatment services (43,53,92,124,317,326). The terms commonly used in the literature to refer to treatment failure—noncompliance or nonadherence—reflect a primary focus on the patient's willingness to follow treatment instructions, generally without specific consideration of whether such treatment is actually available, feasible, appropriate, or affordable. With a few recent exceptions, (cited below) there have been no critical assessments of TB control programs themselves regarding the provision of adequate resources, expertise, and coordination for effective treatment delivery available. Similarly, little systematic information exists on successful TB control programs responsible for high rates of treatment completion.

Nevertheless, greater examination of past experience with TB control and the broader service delivery issues will be needed to fully address the problem of how to reduce rates of TB in the future and, particularly, to avoid further generation of MDR-TB. The issue of treatment failure has immediate repercussions for patients with active TB and their communities. It is most likely to be the focus of future efforts to control the disease. In particular, the ability of a program to effectively supervise treatment such as in directly observed treatment (DOT) may depend, in part, on the quality of its overall management and organization (46).

Because of inadequacies in the information base, it is not feasible in this chapter to review all the relevant issues regarding treatment failure in the same detail or to capture all of their important specifics. However, it is possible to make some preliminary comments about the nature of the problem and about potential causes of treatment failure, if only to provide a general framework for subsequent study. Discussed below are a number of overlapping and interrelated issues relevant to treatment outcome, grouped into the following general categories: availability and quality of TB control services; prescription of optimal treatment regimens; and personal behavioral characteristics influencing completion of treatment. The relative importance of each of the factors in the overall problem cannot be assessed at present with the available data.

Provision of TB Control Services

All States delegate overall responsibility for controlling the spread of TB and other communicable diseases to State and local health agencies, most of which, in turn, contract with local hospitals and clinics to provide TB services. Statutes enacted by State legislatures provide both mandatory and discretionary authorities concerning the conduct of TB control in each State. Although the specific terms of these authorities vary among States, common elements include the ability to order medical examination of individuals suspected of having active TB, to deliver treatment, and, if necessary, use a range of public health powers to impose such treatment or to detain and isolate infectious individuals. A recent analysis of State TB laws concluded that the majority of such statutes are antiquated and may be incompatible with current standards of constitutional law and public health. Such laws include many of those concerning the way in which health officials determine whether an individual poses a significant risk to the public's health, whether the individual has a right to a fair hearing, and whether health officials should be required to try less restrictive measures before imposing more restrictive ones in order to impose compulsory treatment (124). In general, these statutes focus on specifying the circumstances in which health officials can compel an infectious individual to receive treatment, rather than specifying the public health requirements and objectives of a publicly funded TB control system.

There is little systematic information on how State and local programs have carried out their statutory authorities regarding TB control in recent years. Preliminary results of a recent CDC survey of TB control laws and regulations (conducted independently of the one cited above) indicate that State programs differ in basic approaches to TB control. CDC's survey found variations in services designed to assure that patients are treated until cured and in services for monitoring treatment (such as hospital discharge planning) (336). CDC is currently drafting recommendations that States can use in improving their TB control laws and regulations, in an effort to enhance the quality and uniformity of TB control services across the country.

Although States have broad public health powers to order treatment and detention, if deemed necessary, for patients with active TB, they are not legally required to assure that patients are treated until cured. Communicable disease statutes generally limit the scope of that authority to the point of ensuring that patients are rendered noninfectious (which may well be temporary if treatment is not continued until completion) (9).

Nevertheless, completion of treatment is one of the primary goals of TB control, despite the absence of a specific legal responsibility for it. In practice, health departments and TB control programs are responsible for a variety of TB services (some of which are uniquely public health activities), although not all programs provide all of these services listed below:

- surveillance (maintaining registries of clinical information concerning cases and suspected cases and conducting contact investigations to locate additional cases);
- containment (screening for tuberculous infection, diagnosis and treatment of active disease, and preventive treatment);
- purchasing supplies of anti-TB drugs;
- education (professional, public, and patient-oriented);
- laboratory services for diagnosis and drug susceptibility testing;
- medical consultation for primary care providers treating TB patients; and
- followup services (e.g., supervising treatment delivery, including rapid detection and response to evidence of treatment interruption or failure), and coordinating social assistance, substance abuse treatment, or housing services for patients (92).

It is widely held, though infrequently documented, that public health services in the United States have generally not kept pace with health problems in recent years, resulting in part from dwindling resources, lack of expertise, and outdated technologies (12,146). Similarly, serious problems in TB control programs have been noted, including a decline in public funding, lack of access to outpatient TB treatment services and supportive services (such as substance abuse treatment, social assistance, mental health care, and stable housing), and problems maintaining followup of patients on treatment (45,46,83,90,240). In addition, numerous aspects of clinic management that present practical obstacles to care (such as long waiting times, an inhospitable environment for personal care, and lack of flexible service hours, etc.) have been discussed (92).

Thus far, the critiques reporting serious problems have focused on New York City's TB services; detailed accounts of such services elsewhere are absent from the literature, even though similar types of problems are believed to exist in other areas, both urban and rural. CDC's two recent major initiatives, the 1989 Strategic Plan for the Elimination of TB and the 1992 National Action Plan to Combat MDR-TB (see chapter 7) were aimed, in part, at correcting common deficiencies in State and local TB control services (in addition to refocusing and reinvigorating Federal involvement in TB control). The extent to which States have addressed the issues locally, by adopting their own plans to control TB and by supporting high-quality services, are not well documented.[3]

Medical Care Practices

Practicing physicians play a direct role in the outcome of treatment for TB patients in several ways, the most obvious of which is the prescription of an optimal regimen of anti-TB drugs. Related to this is the ability to diagnose the disease promptly and accurately, and to report and record susceptibility testing results. Patients' immunosuppression (due to HIV or other conditions) increase the practical difficulties physicians face in diagnosing TB (see chapter 5).

Closure of many of the specialized facilities for treating TB in the 1960s and 1970s has gradually shifted the job of TB diagnosis and treatment to primary care physicians, many of whom, even in high TB prevalence areas, are unaccustomed to seeing patients with active TB or MDR-TB. As a result, physicians may be less likely to suspect TB, to diagnose it quickly, and to prescribe the most efficacious treatment regimens (or to refer to others with greater expertise) (241). Practical limitations of confirmatory testing to verify the diagnosis may add to these difficulties (92). A critical mistake physicians can make is to add a single drug at a time to a failing regimen; patients treated this way have been found to develop drug resistance sequentially to each additional agent (116,153,366).

A 1983 survey of patients who developed TB again after a course of treatment documented prescribing errors by physicians in the failure of previous treatment. The survey, including 800 patients reported as having recurrent TB disease in 23 health jurisdictions nationwide, found that many of the patients were prescribed inadequate or inappropriate treatment with regard to choice of drugs, dosage, and/or duration for their original episode of TB. In addition, the survey found physicians in private practice were more likely to make these mistakes than physicians in other types of practices (such as health departments) (173).

Additional data on the extent and nature of prescribing errors in TB treatment recently became available from a CDC-sponsored survey of 1,772 physicians in public and private practice, including both generalists and specialists (318). Using a mailed questionnaire, the survey was assigned to determine the extent of physician awareness of CDC and American Thoracic Society guidelines on recommended treatment regimens and the extent that physicians would prescribe efficacious treatment regimens as specified in those guidelines. Preliminary results of the survey suggested that only about 58 percent of the physicians, when asked how they would treat a hypothetical patient with active TB, specified one of the recommended regimens. Specialists or those with fewer years in practice were more likely than generalists or those with more years in practice to describe a recommended regimen.

Another way in which physicians can influence the outcome of treatment is by assuming at least partial responsibility for ensuring that patients take the prescribed treatment continuously and completely (155,265,266). In certain areas, responsibility for monitoring patients on treatment is shared with, or completely delegated to, staff

---

3 Through State reports and funding applications, CDC collects some of this information, and reports it in its quarterly publication for public health departments, *TB Notes*, but has not published it for general review.)

from the local TB control program—nurse case managers or outreach workers (92). In other areas, there may be no standard procedure in place to follow patients' progress with treatment, a carry-over from the privatization of TB care that followed the closure of sanatoria and most specialized TB clinics in the 1960s and 1970s and their incorporation into general medical practice (153).

Patient Behavior

In cases where an optimal combination of anti-TB drugs is prescribed, available, and feasible for the patient to take for the entire period of time, success of treatment ultimately hinges on patients taking their medication according to schedule. In practice, this also requires that the patient regularly submit sputum samples (so that progress with treatment can be measured) and that the patient regularly picks up medication supplies and keeps to a schedule of appointments with the health care provider responsible for delivering and monitoring the treatment. Aside from the small proportion of patients who refuse treatment under any circumstances or who are mentally or psychologically unable to follow a course of treatment, the bulk of the available evidence suggests that most patients would complete treatment if it were feasible to do so or if encouraged to do so through progressively more stringent measures (43,149), as allowed by law to protect the public health.

The medical literature pertaining to patients' willingness and ability to follow an entire course of TB treatment dates back to the 1950s, when it was noted that many hospitalized patients who were given their TB medication at the bedside still did not actually take it and that only about half of patients on outpatient treatment took their medication (266,269). Since then, the issue of patient noncompliance or nonadherence, as it is generally referred to, has been extensively reviewed, most notably over the years by Sbarbaro and in a recent comprehensive review by Sumartojo (266,317). These and other reviews of the role of patient behavior in the success of TB treatment suggest that the relevant context for such behavior encompasses factors both within and beyond a patient's control.

In some cases, a variety of social, economic, and cultural factors, such as homelessness, substance abuse, financial barriers to medical care or general poverty in general, and unfamiliarity with or distrust of Western medical care, may be very relevant to patients' behavior toward TB treatment (95,263,317). In other cases, none of the above may apply. Etkind and colleagues cite examples of a physician at a local teaching hospital in Massachusetts who would not complete his own treatment regimen and of a working corporate executive who had active TB for 4 years and developed MDR-TB as a result of erratic drug-taking (94). One expert noted that the majority of newly diagnosed cases of TB occur among "just plain folks" i.e., individuals with no apparent social or behavioral characteristic(s) that would suggest that he or she is likely to take the medication erratically or not at all (149).

Not surprisingly, researchers have been unable to identify a set of patient characteristics that would permit reliable predictions of patients who will complete treatment with little or no encouragement and those who will fail treatment even with extraordinary amounts of assistance (317). To some extent, this naturally complex behavior may be difficult to simplify to a set of predictive traits. Given the nature of the treatment regimen, it may be reasonable to assume that many, if not most, patients could encounter difficulties staying the course, but that those with major problems, such as homelessness or mental illness, would be more likely to fail treatment without special assistance or residential care (94,271). The most difficult practical issue in this regard concerns the majority of patients without such major problems whose behavior toward the treatment regimen cannot be reliably predicted.

AVAILABLE STRATEGIES FOR IMPROVING TREATMENT DELIVERY

As discussed above, the outcome of TB treatment may be determined by a number of interrelated factors concerning the organization and quality of services, the prescription of an optimal regimen, and the behavior of patients. Accordingly, strategies to improve the chances of cure following treatment may need to involve several types of changes in treatment delivery. Although these changes can be guided by Federal recommendations such as those developed by CDC's Advisory Council for the Elimination of Tuberculosis), the actual decisions about the nature and extent of such changes in treatment delivery will be made by State and local health officials, based in part on available resources and expertise, social and cultural characteristics of the patient population, and available medical services.

Current methods of treatment delivery in the United States can be characterized as heterogeneous, encompassing self-administered (unsupervised) treatment, various degrees of supervision, and even involuntary commitment with compulsory treatment. During the past several decades, self-administered treatment has generally been the norm. Treatment is delivered in many different types of sites, including general outpatient clinics, chest clinics, correctional facilities, private medical practices, hospitals, and long-term care facilities (92).

A number of strategies for improving treatment delivery are currently being considered and debated among health officials, community groups, and policymakers. Many of these are already being used to some extent in some areas. These strategies include:

- greater use of combination medications, such as Rifamate™ (INH and RIF) or a three-drug combination, Rifater™ (INH, RIF, and PZA), which is expected to be commercially available in the United States in 1993.
- greater use of intermittent regimens, rather than daily regimens, which make direct observation of treatment feasible on a wider scale.
- greater use of DOT, either in a treatment facility or in the community, conducted by health care workers or outreach workers.
- greater attention to followup of each case, by public health nurses or outreach workers, involving planning for continuation of treatment and referral to other health and social services after patient discharge such as treatment for substance abuse, HIV treatment, stable housing, mental health services.
- use of incentives, as appropriate, including provision of money, bus tokens, food, or individually determined "gifts" to encourage sustained participation in treatment.
- administrative changes in clinic operations, such as reduced waiting times, appointment reminders, followup of missed appointments, weekend hours.
- use of residential or long-term treatment facilities, as necessary.
- improved professional training for TB diagnosis and treatment.
- educational programs for patients and the community at large.

An adequate public health approach for improving the delivery of TB treatment would likely involve some or all of these strategies, and perhaps others as well, depending on local needs and conditions. In the long run, the ability of TB control programs to implement these strategies will depend on consistent funding provided by the State or Federal Government and the quality of each program's organization, management, and expertise. Inevitably in some areas, strategies designed to assist patients in completing TB treatment will also address problems such as acquired immunodeficiency virus (AIDS), substance abuse, homelessness, and mental illness.

A central issue in improving outcomes of TB treatment concerns the degree to which supervision by HCWs is necessary to bring about higher rates of treatment completion. Much of the recent policy debate about TB control at national and local levels has focused on this issue. Although supervised treatment was recommended by experts long ago, and has been used extensively in other countries for many years, it has been used to only a limited extent in the United States (193, 266,273). CDC estimated that in 1991, approximately 17 percent of TB patients (approximately 4,400) were receiving treatment under direct observation. Two-thirds of this was paid for by CDC cooperative agreement funds employing 213 outreach workers (370). In 1991, $8.5 million was awarded through 46 TB cooperative agreements to 34 States, the District of Columbia, Puerto Rico, Guam, and nine major U.S. cities. In New York City, approximately 500 patients are currently receiving directly observed treatment regimens, and this number is expected to double by the end of 1993 (130). Only three States' statutes (Maine, Michigan, and Minnesota) explicitly provide for DOT as a routine service (124).

CDC defines DOT as observation of the patient by a health care provider or another responsible person (who has frequent contact with the patient, such as family members, social workers, or clergy) as the patient ingests anti-TB medications (366). Some programs limit DOT to health care facilities, which require that the patient visit the facility 2 or 3 times a week. In other areas, workers go out into the community, meeting patients at their residence or at another site (366). DOT can rarely be offered by private physicians without assistance from the local health department because private practices generally do not employ staff to perform this function (43). Although simple in concept, DOT is a labor-intensive effort in practice, requiring skill, diligence, and perseverance on the part of outreach workers (43,266). Furthermore, in some populations, its effectiveness may depend on the simultaneous use of other interventions, such as provision of methadone treatment and on the use of field workers familiar with the practical issues of working with individuals with AIDS and those who use intravenous drugs (68).

Expert groups have recently recommended more widespread use of DOT for most patients with TB, particularly those with resistance to one or more of the first-line drugs (157,366). CDC recommended that all patients be considered for DOT, but that local decisions regarding the expanded use of DOT should be based on completion rates for each area. A report by the United Hospital Fund, which focused on TB control issues in New York City, went further by recommending mandatory DOT for all patients; this would remain in effect until there was convincing evidence mounted in each case showing treatment was longer needed (83).

Critics argue that requiring all patients' treatment be directly observed is "wasteful, inefficient, and gratuitously annoying" and "undercuts the legitimate desire to individualize treatment and to use the least restrictive and intrusive public health interventions" (9). Moreover, it is argued that other interventions, such as effective discharge planning and provision of stable housing, can also increase completion rates without DOT, although close followup of patients' progress would be needed to judge when DOT would become necessary (9). Others hold that universal, mandatory DOT would be a violation of individual liberty and would create undue burden on those who can complete treatment without it; accordingly, it is argued, DOT should be imposed only after an administrative or judicial hearing in each case to determine whether the patient has not taken treatment or is at high risk of taking treatment erratically or not at all (83).

Several programs have described high completion rates among patients treated under direct observation (92). In Denver, where DOT has been used for many years for patients on intermittent regimens, more than 90 percent of patients complete treatment (61). Even higher rates were reported in South Carolina, where the health department routinely uses a variety of strategies, including DOT (and even court-ordered DOT, when necessary) (354). There are also several examples in the literature on programs in which patients who have previously failed treatment were successfully treated under direct observation (187,272). Recent data on results of DOT in Mississippi suggests that TB case rates leveled off and then, after DOT was expanded to include over 90 percent of cases on treatment, began to decline (139). Some populations may be difficult to reach even through DOT: a recent report cited data indicating that among individuals using crack cocaine, DOT alone was not particularly successful in increasing treatment completion rates (349).

While these descriptive studies suggest that DOT may work under certain circumstances and not in others, the effectiveness of DOT compared with other strategies or among broader populations has not yet been examined in prospective, controlled studies. The cost-effectiveness of DOT compared with other strategies is similarly unknown. Comparisons between the cost of treating a patient under DOT versus the cost of treating a patient with MDR-TB are not relevant for public policy discussions since not all patients treated without DOT develop MDR-TB and not all patients on DOT are assured of cure (157). A more complete assessment of costs and outcomes is needed to generate useful information.

In general, improvement in delivery of TB treatment will require the availability of several different treatment strategies that can be applied according to local needs and customs, levels of community involvement, and amounts of public health resources. As a public health strategy, unsupervised treatment appears to be an inadequate approach to control TB and to prevent MDR-TB, even though some patients may succeed without supervision. More active involvement by public health workers in each patient's course of treatment would appear necessary in many areas, along with improved educational efforts for physicians concerning the prescription of optimal TB treatment. The adoption of a comprehensive system of services and support may be a valuable objective for many programs. As described by Sumartojo, such a comprehensive system would include: teams of HCWs responsible for continuity of care, careful case management and followup, clinical TB services that are accessible and acceptable to patients, social assistance provided to patients who need it, and supervision of treatment (317). Ongoing evaluation of effectiveness of treatment will be needed to make judgments about long-term changes in the delivery of TB treatment.

Federal Involvement in Tuberculosis Control and Research 7

Primary responsibility for designing and carrying out tuberculosis (TB) control services in the United States rests not with Federal officials, but with State public health departments and local health authorities. Governed by State laws that specify overall responsibilities regarding TB and the use of public health powers intended to prevent further transmission of the disease (124), State public health departments provide and coordinate a range of services. To varying degrees, these services generally include: surveillance; laboratory services, treatment, and followup; contact investigation; education; and consultation (93).

Private health care providers and a variety of organized groups (e.g., patient advocacy groups, public and professional groups, voluntary organizations, and community-based organizations) are also closely involved in these activities. In practice, individual TB control programs differ substantially from place to place, according to available resources, quality of the program management, available expertise, local prevalence of the disease, and characteristics of the affected population.

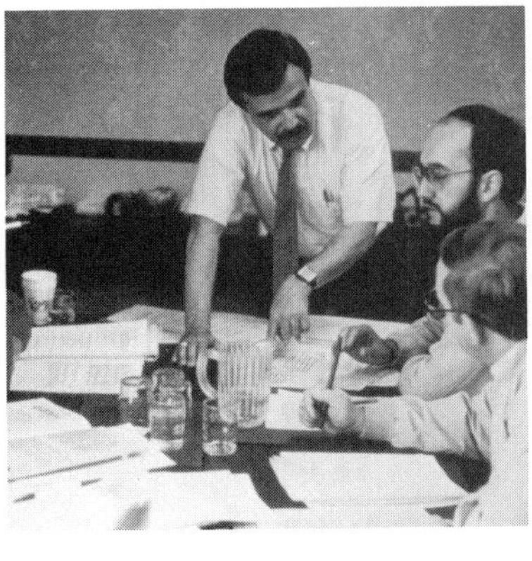

In the United States, the Federal Government is responsible for developing a national plan to control TB and for assisting in various ways to implement it. Although the Federal Government has long held responsibilities in regard to TB control (see box 7-A), the resurgence of TB has recently prompted Federal agencies and departments to expand their involvement, particularly in guidance and oversight of prevention and treatment activities, support of research and development, and assuring the availability of anti-TB drugs. In addition, the increasing size of the patient population has implications for reimbursement of TB services through government-sponsored health insurance programs like Medicaid and Medicare.

Box 7-A—The History of Tuberculosis Prevention and Control Within the U.S. Public Health Service

From the late 1800s to the 1940s, the primary method of tuberculosis (TB) control was the isolation of infected individuals in special sanatoriums until death or until the disease went into remission. In the early part of this century, TB control was largely a voluntary grass-roots movement at the State and local level. Local health departments set up TB programs at the urging of the Society for the Prevention of Tuberculosis, which had been established in 1904. With the advent of antibiotics in the 1940s, effective treatment for TB became possible. The U.S. Public Health Service's (PHS) Bureau of State Services became involved in the evaluation of anti-tuberculosis drugs such as streptomycin, para-amino salicyclic acid, and isoniazid both in the United States and Europe. During the 1940s and 1950s, TB treatment still involved a long stay in a sanatorium with additional treatment and lifelong followup after discharge.

In 1944 Congress passed the Public Health Service Act, which established the Division of Tuberculosis Control within PHS and authorized grants to States for tuberculosis control. By the end of World War II, PHS had organized TB support teams available to population centers with more than 100,000 residents to augment the supply of x-ray and case finding staff. By 1953, these teams had examined about 20 million people in 20 cities. Better living conditions and the availability of drugs to treat TB led to a decrease in the number of new cases found by the support teams. This decrease along with rising costs and growing concern about exposure to x-rays led PHS to discontinue the program.

As it became obvious by the 1960s that long-term isolation of patients with active disease was not necessary to protect the patient and the community, PHS began to recommend that States close their sanatoriums and treat patients mainly on an outpatient basis. Although this change represented significant potential savings to State and local governments, the closing of sanatoriums also placed new demands on local health departments to conduct followup of TB patients. In the early 1960s, health department case registers carried 75,000 to 100,000 TB patients requiring outpatient followup services. In addition, health departments also had to identify, test, and possibly treat an average of five individuals that each case of active TB may have infected. These new demands on local health departments necessitated assistance from PHS.

In 1959, TB experts met in Harriman, New York to take stock of the Nation's TB control efforts and to develop standards for evaluating control programs. This meeting came to be known as the Arden House

This chapter focuses on the current involvement of the Federal Government in public health efforts to control TB, research and development of new technologies for diagnosis and treatment of TB, regulation of TB treatment interventions, health services research, and reimbursement for TB services. The discussion is based mainly on information obtained by the Office of Technology Assessment (OTA) from each agency, institute, or organization. OTA received information that contained varying degrees of detail and synthesis regarding each group's involvement in TB-related work. Rather than attempting to provide a detailed account or evaluation of all Federal activities directly or indirectly related to TB, the discussion that follows highlights the major current initiatives and programs concerning TB and the approximate funding allocated for them. The discussion provides recent spending information for the few agencies able to distinguish TB money from other funds.

PUBLIC HEALTH ACTIVITIES

The Centers for Disease Control and Prevention

The lead agency for TB control operations within the Federal Government is the Centers for Disease Control and Prevention (CDC). In fiscal year 1993 CDC's budget for TB control activities totaled approximately $79 million: $34.3 million in project grants to State and local health departments in support of prevention and control

Conference. The group recommended eradication of TB mainly through drug treatment. A set of 11 secondary recommendations focused on making treatment feasible and efficient, led to the current approach to TB prevention and control—to treat active disease in order to cure the patient and prevent further spread of infection in order to prevent the development of active disease.

On November 1, 1960, the Tuberculosis Branch of the PHS's Bureau of State Services was organizationally transferred to the then Communicable Disease Center (CDC). In 1960, the Branch also initiated Federal TB project grants to State and local governments in response to the Surgeon General's Task Force on Tuberculosis. Funding for these grants reached a peak of $20 million in 1968. In addition to providing funds, the CDC's TB missions have been to provide national leadership in the development and implementation of effective strategies to interrupt the transmission of TB and ultimately eliminate the disease. CDC has established policies and guidelines for TB control programs in conjunction with American Thoracic Society. A important function of CDC has been to gather data on the disease to define the overall tuberculosis problem and examine more specific issues. CDC has provided consultative visits by headquarters staff to local programs and in some areas direct long-term assignments of CDC staff have been made to assist in program implementation. In addition, the agency provides training courses for TB workers.

During the late 1960s, categorical TB project grants were phased out in favor of General Public Health Formula Grants under section 314(d)of the Public Health Service Act (Ch. 373, 58 Stat. 682). Because these new grants did not require that State and local governments use any of the funds for TB control, many health departments redistributed the funds to other purposes.

Uniform nationwide reporting of active TB cases to CDC began in 1953. For the next three decades, the United States saw a decline in active TB cases, from 84,304 reported in 1953 to a low of 22,255 cases in 1984. After 1985, however, the number of new cases began to increase again to 26,673 in 1992. Despite the overall increasing morbidity, in much of the country, TB had retreated into well-defined segments of the population (see chapter 3). Against this background and as a result of the occurrence of outbreaks of drug-resistant TB, CDC coordinated the 1988 "Strategic Plan for the Elimination of Tuberculosis in the United States" and the 1992 "National Action Plan to Combat Multidrug-Resistant Tuberculosis" described in chapter 7.

SOURCE: C. Bozzi, Assistant to the Director for Tuberculosis Coordination, Division of TB Elimination, Centers for Disease Control and Prevention, Public Health Service, U.S. Department of Health and Human Services, Atlanta, GA, personal communication, 1993.

services (including directly observed therapy (DOT) and educational activities); $39.2 million in emergency funds appropriated separately by Congress for TB control programs in six States and seven cities most heavily affected by TB; and $5.2 million for TB program operations at CDC. In addition to the $79 million designated for TB, $25.4 million designated for human immunodeficiency virus (HIV) activities were used for HIV-related TB activities (e.g., investigation of MDR-TB outbreaks and related issues; expansion of screening and prevention demonstration projects in drug treatment centers, correctional facilities, and other sites; and expansion of demonstration projects for the treatment and prevention of TB in HIV-infected or at-risk populations) (255, 330). Table 7-1 gives a breakdown of CDC TB spending in fiscal year 1993 according to the use to which the funds are put.

The total expenditure for fiscal year 1993 greatly exceeded previous years' budgets (see figure 7-1). For fiscal year 1994, the President requested that Congress appropriate $129 million for TB control at the U.S. Department of Health and Human Services (U.S. DHHS); the $50 million increase over 1993 is intended to support State programs in directly observed therapy and screening in high-risk populations, and to improve TB diagnosis, surveillance, prevention, and education (332).

The American Lung Association (ALA), a voluntary, national organization originally founded

Table 7-1—U.S. Centers for Disease Control and Prevention Spending for Tuberculosis by Function, Fiscal Year 1993

	Dollars ($ millions)	Percent of budget
Community-based control programs (screening, treatment, prevention, infection control)	$ 36.9	35%
Outreach and service linkage (implementation of directly observed therapy)	36.7	35
Research and demonstration	9.8	9
Surveillance, epidemiology and data systems	7.0	7
Laboratory services	4.8	5
Public education and information	4.4	4
Professional competence assurance (training for service providers, physicians, researchers, and laboratory personnel)	2.2	2
Leadership and administration (technical assistance to improve management of State and local TB control programs)	2.2	2
Community protection/regulatory programs	NA	NA
Total	$104.0	100%[a]

NA = not available.

[a] Component percentages do not add up to 100 percent due to rounding error.

SOURCE: Office of Technology Assessment, 1993, based on data from C. Bozzi, Assistant to the Director for Tuberculosis Coordination, Division of Tuberculosis Elimination, Public Health Service, Centers for Disease Control and Prevention, U.S. Department of Health and Human Services, Atlanta, GA, personal communication, July 9, 1993.

in 1904 to coordinate public and private TB control campaigns (262), recently recommended that CDC's budget for TB control be increased to $380 million in fiscal year 1994, stating that additional funds are needed to support DOT, training and educational activities, surveillance and epidemiologic studies, and evaluation of current programs (244).

ALA also recommended that continued funding to the States through CDC's project grants be contingent on the adoption of an adequate State TB elimination plan (244). Other experts have suggested additional uses for CDC's TB funds, including direct support of clinical services (as in New York City chest clinics of the 1970s) and the facilities in which they are housed, regional "centers of excellence" specializing in the care of patients with TB, long-term care facilities and subsidized housing for TB patients, and bulk purchasing of anti-TB drugs and infection control supplies (130).

The CDC's Division of TB Elimination had its organizational beginnings in the 1940s. Box 7-A gives a history of U.S. Public Health Service (PHS) involvement in TB control. Federal TB activities and funding were drastically scaled back in the late 1960s as TB was perceived to be under control, but were restarted in the early 1980s (240). In the mid-1980s, following indications that TB was no longer in decline and that a resurgence in cases was likely, CDC developed a comprehensive plan for TB control, entitled "A Strategic Plan for the Elimination of Tuberculosis in the United States." The plan was adopted in 1988, endorsed by then U.S. DHHS Secretary Louis Sullivan, and set as a national goal the elimination of TB by the year 2010 (i.e., reducing its incidence to less than one in a million).

Figure 7-1—Tuberculosis Funding, U.S. Centers for Disease Control and Prevention, Fiscal Years 1960-93

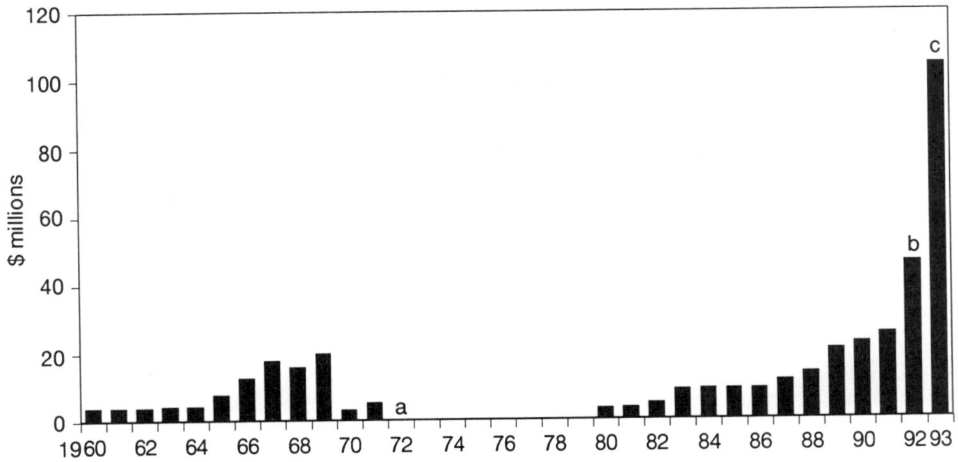

a Fiscal years 1972 through 1982 categorical grants ceased. Funds to States were in block grants not specific for TB.
b Fiscal year 1992 includes $26 million in HIV funds used for HIV-related TB activities.
c Fiscal year 1993 includes $25 million in HIV funds used for HIV-related TB activities.

SOURCE: Office of Technology Assessment, 1993, based on data from the Department of Health and Human Services, Public Health Service, Centers for Disease Control and Prevention.

The plan also set a target of 3.5 cases per 100,000 population by the year 2000 as an interim goal. To achieve this, the plan emphasized three concurrent efforts: more intensive use of existing prevention and control methods; the development and evaluation of new diagnostic, treatment, and prevention technologies; and the rapid transfer of knowledge, skills, and new technologies into clinical and public health practice (270,367).

Shortly thereafter, CDC, together with the American Thoracic Society and representatives from 22 national organizations, coordinated the National Tuberculosis Training Initiative, an educational effort geared toward medical and allied health professionals. The initiative's purpose was to make medical and public health professionals aware of the Strategic Plan, to improve the quality of care for individuals with tuberculous infection and active disease, and to improve medical education regarding TB (239). Through this effort, U.S. DHHS published the "Core Curriculum on Tuberculosis," summarizing current information on TB and TB control (378).

In 1992, following the recent worsening of the problem as indicated by the series of MDR-TB outbreaks, CDC released another national plan designed to complement and enhance the Strategic Plan: the "National Action Plan to Combat Multidrug-Resistant Tuberculosis" (363). The Action Plan was developed by a task force assembled by CDC, composed of representatives from a number of Federal agencies, and consultants from various other public health groups. The task force's main focus was to define ways of intervening rapidly to prevent further transmission and generation of drug-resistant TB, as part of its ongoing efforts to control TB in general. The Action Plan identified a series of objectives in TB control and laid out a detailed plan of implementation involving an array of Government agencies and professional organizations with ongoing responsibilities in TB control and research. In general, the Action Plan defined a process to bring the current outbreaks under

Box 7-B—A Summary of the U.S. Centers for Disease Control and Prevention's Multidrug-Resistant Tuberculosis Action Plan

In response to the emergence of MDR-TB, a Federal task force was convened in December 1991 to develop a national action plan to combat the problem. The plan identifies a number of objectives to be undertaken at the national level. The objectives [as described by CDC staff in a recent article] are summarized [here:]

Epidemiology and Surveillance—To better define the magnitude and nature of MDR-TB, national surveillance will be expanded to capture information on the incidence of drug-resistant TB. Epidemiologic studies will be used to identify where MDR-TB is being spread, what activities are associated with increases or decreases in transmission, and which preventive strategies are effective in community and in institutional settings. The impact of HIV infection on recent trends in TB disease and infection, including MDR-TB, will be assessed.

Laboratory Diagnosis—To improve the rapidity, sensitivity, and reliability of diagnostic methods for MDR-TB, widespread changes and improvements need to be implemented in clinical and public health laboratories. These changes include the use of the most sensitive and rapid laboratory diagnostic methods available, including the use of a primary susceptibility test panel of five drugs (INH, RIF, PZA, ethambutol, and streptomycin). New equipment, training courses, and information systems will be used in laboratories to achieve these objectives.

Patient Management—Activities need to be implemented to prevent patients with drug-susceptible TB from developing drug-resistant disease and to manage patients optimally who have developed drug-resistant disease. To achieve these goals, effective initial anti-tuberculosis therapy regimens and implementation of DOT [directly observed treatment] for all TB patients who would benefit from it, regardless of their ability to pay for these services, will be promoted. Options for the long-term hospitalization of drug-resistant TB patients, when needed, will be explored. Efforts to facilitate access to diagnosis and treatment will be directed to those at high risk for both TB and nonadherence to therapy, such as persons who are homeless, mobile populations of migrant farm workers, refugees and immigrants from areas with a high prevalence of TB, and persons with substance abuse problems.

Screening and Preventive Therapy—To distinguish persons who are infected or at risk of developing MDR-TB to help prevent them from developing clinically active TB, widespread dissemination and

control, to prevent new ones, and to resume progress toward elimination of TB (see box 7-B summarizing key points of the MDR Action Plan).

CDC estimates that full implementation of those parts of the Action Plan for which it has responsibility would require $380 million in annual spending (1993 dollars) above the $104 million spent in fiscal year 1993. Estimates from other agencies are not available, but CDC has begun collecting such information following OTA's queries.

In an effort to help OTA assess CDC's priorities in implementing its part of the Action Plan should Congress not fully fund the Action Plan in a single year, CDC supplied OTA with its estimates of how it would allocate funding increases of $50 million, $95 million, and the full $380 million above fiscal year 1993 levels. CDC gave these funding breakdowns according to the same categories presented in table 7-1. CDC's projections indicate that for these three potential funding levels, the proportion of funds allocated to each spending category would be essentially the same as that for actual fiscal year 1993 funding; partial or full funding would not change CDC's relative priorities among these funding categories (38). No information on priorities within each spending category was available to OTA[1]

[1] CDC has also identified 215 individual steps necessary to implement the Action Plan, assigning each a priority score of "1" (highest priority), "2", or "3" (lowest priority) (369). The vast majority of implentation steps were given a priority of "1" (76 percent) with most of the rest (23 percent) given the middle score of "2." Although these priorities underscore the sense of urgency of the Federal interagency group that prepared the Action Plan, they do not indicate how CDC and other agencies would proceed if funding did not permit full implementation of all steps identified as high priority.

implementation of recently published guidelines on management of persons exposed to MDR-TB will be promoted. Screening and preventive therapy (directly observed when necessary) among populations at risk for both TB and nonadherence to therapy will be implemented.

Infection and Outbreak Control—Given the circumstances of recent MDR-TB outbreaks in hospital and correctional institutions, the risk of transmission of MDR-TB to patients, workers, and others in institutional settings needs to be minimized. Implementation of current guidelines for reducing this risk is of the highest priority. Adequate screening and monitoring for TB infection among workers in settings where there is a substantial risk of TB transmission will be ensured.

Outbreaks represent a challenge to public health authorities in controlling TB. Various officials and organizations will collaborate to enhance the control of outbreaks of MDR-TB.

Program Evaluation—TB control programs need to be evaluated for effectiveness in managing patients and preventing the development of MDR-TB. Local epidemiologic data will be used for assessing the adequacy of the TB control programs.

Information Dissemination, Training, and Education—To disseminate information about MDR-TB and its prevention and control, high-risk populations, such as persons working in drug treatment centers, homeless shelters, HIV clinics, and correctional and other institutions with close living quarters, and their clients; refugees; and immigrants will be identified to be educated about TB. A system for the professional education of those involved in the prevention, control, diagnosis, and treatment of TB will be developed.

Research—Research is needed to identify better methods to combat MDR-TB. Increased knowledge of the basic genetics and biology of *M. tuberculosis* is necessary to understanding better the pathogenesis, immune response, and mechanisms of drug resistance of TB, so that improved diagnostic assays, drugs, and vaccines can be developed. A research subcommittee of the Public Health Service's National MDR-TB Task Force was recently formed to coordinate current and future TB research efforts among participating Federal agencies.

SOURCE: Excerpt from M.E. Villarino, L.J. Geiter, and P.M. Simone, "Multi-Drug Resistant Tuberculosis Challenge to Public Health Efforts to Control Tuberculosis," *Public Health Reports* 107(6):623-624, 1992.

As part of its current TB control efforts, the CDC has also encouraged the formation of State and local TB elimination advisory committees. By the end of 1992, such committees have been formed in 28 areas resulting in TB elimination plans for 10 States and 4 cities (370).

In the past several years, the National Institute for Occupational Safety and Health (NIOSH), an agency within CDC, has conducted studies on occupational risks from respiratory exposures to TB, including health hazard evaluations in hospitals, health clinics, correctional facilities, laboratories, drug treatment centers, homeless shelters, and other sites. Also planned is surveillance for TB in workers; development of methods for detecting and measuring airborne particles containing tubercle bacilli; and evaluation of compliance with standard infection control guidelines in occupational settings (34,368). NIOSH recently conducted a risk assessment on the use of personal respiratory protection in preventing transmission of TB in health care facilities (371) (see chapter 4). It has also recently begun additional research on the effectiveness of infection control interventions, including ventilation systems, ultraviolet light, and respirator efficiency (24).

Occupational Health and Safety Administration

The U.S. Department of Labor's Occupational Health and Safety Administration (OHSA) has regulatory and enforcement responsibilities for workplace health and safety. OHSA's recent TB-related activities include the issuance of guidelines to compliance safety and health officers on conducting inspections following a worker's complaint of TB exposure in the workplace, outreach and training for labor, industry, academia, and professional groups, and 20 workplace inspections in response to employee complaints. OSHA is also a lead agency in implementing several steps in the National Action Plan to Combat MDR-TB (108). OSHA's budget for TB-specific activities was approximately $330,000 in fiscal year 1992 and $339,000 in fiscal year 1993 (36).

U.S. Departments of Justice and State

Because Federal law bars immigration of individuals with communicable diseases, including active TB, while they are infectious (8 USC 1182, 1224, 1226), the U.S. Departments of Justice and State also play roles in TB control. Consular officers in U.S. embassies abroad require applicants for immigration visas to undergo chest x-rays and sputum smears (if the chest x-ray is abnormal). Those found to have active TB can usually proceed to the United States once treatment has rendered them noninfectious. At the port of entry, the U.S. Department of Justice's Immigration and Naturalization Service (INS) notifies a CDC quarantine officer who in turn informs State or local health officials in the area the immigrant plans to reside. Consular officers in U.S. embassies abroad can require medical examinations of applicants for nonimmigrant visas as well.

The INS funds detention facilities for individuals found to be in the United States illegally while they await immigration hearings or deportation. At nine of the facilities that the INS runs itself,[2] the PHS Office of Refugee Health provides tuberculin skin tests upon inmates' arrivals with followup diagnosis, treatment of active and latent cases, and notification of relevant State and local health departments for those released in the United States (181). As of July 1, 1993, there were 5,658 persons under INS detention its own and contract facilities (47).

U.S. Department of Veterans Affairs

Through its nationwide system of hospitals, nursing homes, and outpatient clinics, the U.S. Department of Veterans Affairs (U.S. DVA) is responsible for a broad range of TB control services for veterans and their families. In general, the issues faced by these facilities regarding treatment and prevention of TB and the VA's responses to them parallel those outside the VA.

A recent survey found patients with drug-susceptible or drug-resistant TB, some of whom are also HIV-infected, in each of the four U.S. DVA regions of the country (258). In 1992, a cluster of MDR-TB cases was found at one VA medical center, which led to a review by infection control officials of current infection control practices and compliance with existing U.S. DVA guidelines and CDC recommendations for health care facilities (259).

The U.S. DVA reorganized its longstanding infection control program in 1990 under the direction of its Central Office Medical Service, which then issued revised hospital-based infection control guidelines based on recommendations from a number of expert groups. The Medical Service conducts annual infection control surveys, organizes an advisory group on infection control matters within the U.S. DVA, and participates in CDC's national task force on MDR-TB (257). It also coordinates with State health departments in providing TB treatment services, reporting of cases of TB, investigating contacts of cases, and other activities (379). There is no separate budget within the U.S. DVA for TB activities.

---

[2] Some illegal immigrants are detained in facilities run by State governments, local governments, or private firms under contract for the INS. Information on TB services provided to these detainees was not available.

Indian Health Service

The Indian Health Service (IHS) works with State and local health departments to coordinate TB control services for American Indians and Alaska Natives (AI/AN). These services are delivered either through IHS facilities or State health departments. No IHS funds are designated specifically for TB services on a regular basis; however, IHS does provide TB services for special situations as needed (161).

In 1991, 345 cases of TB in individuals self-identified as AI/AN across 33 States were reported to CDC; 86 percent of these cases occurred in children under the age of 5. At least one cluster of TB cases has recently been reported among AI/AN populations—among the Choctaw tribe in Mississippi. In that case, Choctaw representatives requested and received a one-time appropriation of $165,000 from the IHS to upgrade their TB control program. Since 1992, the Mississippi Board of Choctaw has assumed responsibility for developing and implementing its own TB control plan, although the State health department still supplies technical assistance to the tribe (161).

Federal Bureau of Prisons

The Health Services Division of the Federal Bureau of Prisons sets policy concerning TB control within Federal prisons nationwide. As of June 1993, this agency was responsible for just over 78,000 inmates in 71 institutions as well as another 6,000 individuals in less restrictive community-based facilities (186). There is no specific budget for TB services. Beginning in 1990, their policy specified that each prison must maintain a TB control program designed to identify infectious cases, isolate them, and begin effective treatment in accord with CDC guidelines. The basic components of the plan include: chest x-ray, medical history, and physical examination of all incoming inmates; tuberculin skin testing every 2 years; HIV testing for all inmates suspected or known to have active TB; reevaluation of all TB cases at regular intervals; and provisions for all cases that cannot be treated adequately at a given prison site (185,346).

Despite these guidelines, however, experts suggested to OTA that many Federal correctional facilities may not fully comply with these guidelines due to a lack of resources or for other reasons (247,323). OTA found no evidence to determine the extent of compliance with the CDC guidelines among Federal correctional institutions (4,247).

U.S. Agency for International Development

Since being foreign-born is a risk factor for TB in the United States, attempts to control the disease elsewhere in the world may affect the extent of TB here. The U.S. Agency for International Development (U.S. AID), charged with administering the United States' foreign aid to less developed countries, supports TB services and research through several of its health-related programs. TB-related spending has grown in recent years and in 1992 included allocations of:

- $7 million for bacillus Calmette-Guérin (BCG) vaccination of children through the Child Survival program;
- about $850,000 for TB research and analysis, including support for the research and development of a rapid, simple test to diagnose TB appropriate for developing countries; and
- about $500,000 for TB control programs.

Spending for TB control activities includes spending for centrally-administered programs as well as activities carried out by the U.S. Agency for International Development's field missions ranging from direct funding of national TB control programs to funding screening programs carried out by nongovernmental organizations. The agency's HIV/AIDS programs also provide funding to the World Health Organization's Global Program on AIDS that carries out some TB activities related to the problem of dual infection with HIV and TB (196,197).

Health Resources and Services Administration

The Health Resources and Services Administration (HRSA) is an agency of the Public Health Service responsible for supporting health services to disadvantaged and underserved populations as well as improving the education, supply, and distribution of health professionals nationwide. Much of its activities are carried out in cooperation with State and local health departments and private organizations. Although the agency has had no TB-specific budget to-date, the President's budget for fiscal year 1994 includes a $40 million request for such funds. In addition, many of its existing programs support TB activities. HRSA's Bureau of Primary Health Care (BPHC) funds 800 clinics and other grantees who provide primary care including TB screening, diagnostic follow-up, and DOT for individuals at risk of contracting the disease. This includes grantees who receive funding through the Ryan White Comprehensive AIDS Resources Emergency Act (Public Law 101-381). BPHC also currently supports the development of TB educational materials and conferences for health care providers as well as the participation of its primary care programs in clinical trials for those dually infected with HIV and TB. HRSA's Hansen Disease Center in Carville, Louisiana conducts TB drug development research with funds from the CDC and the National Institutes of Health (NIH). In fiscal year 1993, support from CDC and NIH for work at Carville totaled $450,000 with an expected $900,000 for fiscal year 1994 (264).

RESEARCH AND DEVELOPMENT

Although most of the current TB-related research and development is conducted with funds from the NIH, a number of other DHHS offices are also involved. For example, one of the functions of the National Vaccine Program Office (NVPO), which reports to the Assistant Secretary for Health (U.S. DHHS), is to coordinate research carried out through NIH, CDC, the Food and Drug Administration (FDA), and through the U.S. Department of Defense (U.S. DOD), and the Agency for International Development (U.S. AID) on the development and evaluation of vaccines against various diseases (333), including TB. NVPO designated $1.3 million in fiscal year 1992 to support a number of research proposals focusing on the development of effective vaccines for the prevention of TB in immunocompetent and immunocompromised individuals (166). In fiscal year 1993, CDC supported an estimated $9.8 million in TB research and demonstrations that included basic scientific inquiry, behavioral research, new diagnostic tools, infection control, and clinical research into vaccines and treatment (38). The FDA maintains its own research program to aid in the development and evaluation of drugs and other technologies that is charged with regulating.[3] The Substance Abuse and Mental Health Services Administration (SAMHSA) supports some research relevant to the delivery of TB services.

National Institutes of Health

Funding for TB research at NIH has increased substantially in recent years: it went from approximately $300,000 in fiscal year 1985 to $4.3 million in fiscal year 1991, to $15.3 million in fiscal year 1992, to $35.9 million in fiscal year 1993 (37,260). The 1992 budget includes $5.5 million designated for HIV research that was directed to HIV-related TB research; the 1993 budget includes $14.1 million in such HIV money as well as another $4.8 million in one-time funds transferred by the NIH director from her discretionary budget (261).[4] An additional $10.5 mil-

---

[3] The FDA's regulatory responsibilities are described later in this chapter.

[4] HIV funding relevant to TB is counted in NIH's estimates of both its TB funding and its HIV/AIDS spending.

lion was requested in the President's proposed fiscal year 1994 budget for TB research at NIH (332). NIH's TB research agenda covers a broad array of strategies (374):

- Basic research on the molecular biology of tubercle bacilli and immunologic responses to tuberculous infection considered essential for the development of improved treatments, vaccines, and diagnostic methods;
- Studies on the epidemiology and natural history of TB;
- Development of tools to diagnose tuberculous infection and active disease, and to determine drug susceptibility;
- New treatments for drug-susceptible and drug-resistant TB and new delivery methods for these drugs;
- Evaluation of ways to improve patient compliance with treatment;
- Clinical trials of preventive treatment in HIV-infected, purified protein derivative-positive individuals;
- Development of new vaccines to prevent TB;
- Training of new TB researchers (e.g., in career development awards) and improvements in medical education regarding TB;
- Educational efforts geared toward health care workers, patients, and the general public concerning prevention of TB.

In addition, NIH is spending $2.3 million to convert one of its buildings into a specialized laboratory facility for researchers to conduct safe experiments using drug-resistant strains of tubercle bacilli. As part of its requested increase in fiscal year 1994, NIH (through the National Institute for Allergy and Infectious Diseases, (NIAID)) plans to fund one or more "TB Prevention and Control Research Units," multidisciplinary research centers with expertise and activities in epidemiology, basic science, and clinical interventions (260).

Seventeen of the relatively independent institutes and centers that constitute NIH report ongoing TB research or training; NIAID receives the bulk of NIH's budget for TB (57 percent in fiscal year 1993) (376). Among the other 16 institutes and centers involved in TB research and training, those with the largest efforts are the National Center for Research Resources (NCRR), the National Heart, Lung, and Blood Institute (NHLBI), the National Institute for Environmental Health Sciences, the National Institute on Drug Abuse (NIDA), the National Institute of Mental Health (NIMH), the National Center for Nursing Research (NCNR), and the National Institute for General Medical Sciences (NIGMS) (137,167,228,288,314,372,375)).

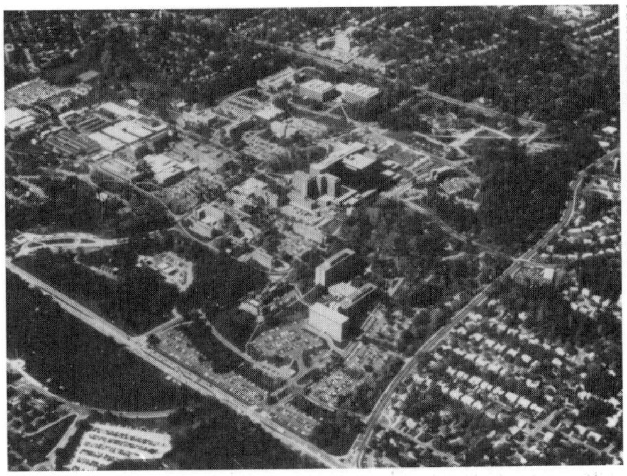

NATIONAL INSTITUTES OF HEALTH

Aerial view of the NIH campus in Bethesda, Maryland. Seventeen of the institutes and centers that constitute NIH support TB-related research and development, although the bulk of this work is funded by the National Institute for Allergy and Infectious Disease.

NIAID participated in the development of TB research strategies for the PHS National Action Plan. The agency estimates that funding for just those Action Plan activities that fall within NIAID's purview would cost $45.6 million in fiscal year 1994, $20.6 million above NIAID's estimated fiscal year 1993 spending for TB and $10.1 million more than the President's requested increase in TB funding for fiscal year 1994 for all of NIH. In spring 1993, an NIH Executive Committee on Tuberculosis Research identified and prioritized new TB research opportunities for all of NIH; complete funding of this research agenda would cost of $102 million above fiscal year 1993 funding.[5]

REGULATION OF TECHNOLOGIES

In its role as regulator of medical drugs and devices, the FDA is responsible for ensuring the safety and effectiveness of the drugs, devices, and diagnostic agents to prevent, detect, and treat TB including BCG and other vaccines, and tuberculin skin tests. Although the agency has no budget specifically for TB-related activities, the FDA's role in TB control in recent years has focused on:

- alleviating the shortage of some anti-TB drugs;
- expediting the approval process for new drugs (e.g., by evaluating their effectiveness with surrogate measures such as early conversion to a negative sputum smear instead of cure rates following the full course of treatment.)
- developing guidelines for assessing the safety and efficacy of new diagnostic devices for rapid detection of TB (e.g. tests using polymerase chain reaction (PCR) technology) as well as devices used to help prevent the spread of *M.tb.* (e.g. germicidal lamps).

Prompted by reports in early 1991 of shortages of some anti-TB drugs and their ingredients, the FDA established a TB task force to examine factors contributing to the problem and to find ways of reestablishing stable supplies. For an interim period, a limited supply of streptomycin (SM) and para-aminosalicylic acid (PAS) was made available through CDC under an investigational new drug agreement for patients with MDR-TB. The FDA is currently working with pharmaceutical manufacturers to resolve problems in the manufacture and sale of anti-TB drugs in the United States and is now attempting to monitor supplies. The agency is also working with companies to encourage the development of implantable forms of anti-TB drugs and combination formulations (121). As mentioned earlier in this chapter, the FDA's regulatory role is complemented by a research program coordinated with the CDC and NIH to aid in the development and evaluation of new diagnostic tools, therapies, and vaccines (226).

HEALTH SERVICES RESEARCH

The U.S. DHHS's Agency for Health Care Policy and Research (AHCPR) shares responsibility for funding research on the effectiveness, appropriateness, and cost of TB health care services and their delivery with CDC and some institutes at NIH. Although most of AHCPR's work is conducted through extramural research grants, it also conducts intramural research and facilitates the development, periodic review, and updating of clinical practice guidelines by panels of experts from outside the Federal government. The agency has had several activities to-date related to TB:

- Supporting the development of guidelines that will include recommendations on screening and prophylactic therapy for TB among HIV-infected people (32);
- Sponsoring educational workshops, such as a seminar for State judges on HIV/AIDS and TB to help them in their adjudication of cases that involve these diseases. Future workshops may be conducted for State legislators, other elected officials, and their staff (221,222);
- Funding ongoing research efforts on HIV/AIDS with an emphasis on studying comorbidities including TB; and
- Working with CDC to develop estimates of costs associated with TB (32).

Research at CDC, especially within its Division of TB Elimination, is increasingly focused on studies of the costs and effectiveness of treatment and other programs related to the control of TB. CDC's increased efforts in this area

[5] This figure includes support for research projects that last for more than 1 year.

are the result of its expertise in TB and its close involvement with the State and local health departments that run TB control programs (191). NIH's research portfolio also contains work relevant to the provision of effective TB health services, particularly behavioral research focusing on treatment compliance (314,375).

HOUSING

The U.S. Department of Housing and Urban Development has no programs specifically targeted to tuberculosis or people with tuberculosis. However, for a short period of time, it did send a representative to the meetings of the CDC-coordinated National MDR-TB Task Force (145).

REIMBURSEMENT FOR TB SERVICES

Disability Programs Administered by the Social Security Administration

The Social Security Administration administers two programs that provide income to disabled individuals. The Social Security Disability Insurance (DI) program pays benefits to disabled individuals who have paid social security taxes and have achieved "insured status" as defined by law. Benefits depend on the amount of taxes paid over a person's career. DI beneficiaries become eligible for Medicare after receiving DI payments for 2 years. The Supplemental Security Income (SSI) program pays benefits to disabled individuals with low-income. SSI pays a standard amount to all beneficiaries and does not require that individuals have paid social security taxes. SSI recipients also become eligible for Medicaid.

Both SSI and DI use the same definition of disability—"an inability to engage in any substantial gainful activity by reason of any physical or mental impairment which can be expected to result in death or which has lasted or can be expected to last for a continuous period of not less than 12 months" (42 USC Sec 423(d)(1)(A) for DI and Sec 1382(a)(3)(A) for SSI). SSA evaluates disability applications in a sequential process to establish that the individual is not engaged in substantial, gainful activity due to an impairment that is listed among SSA's medical impairments or that is at least as severe as a listed impairment. Applicants who do not meet this criteria can also be found to be disabled if they are unable, for at least a year, to do their previous type of work or other generally available work appropriate for their ages, educations, and previous work experiences (88,331).

SSI or DI is not available for most TB patients without other disabling conditions because of the statutory requirement that the patient's impairment last for at least twelve months. As described in earlier chapters, individuals with active, drug-susceptible TB and no other complicating conditions are usually infectious for only the first few weeks of treatment and are likely to be able to work afterwards. Patients with drug-resistant strains may be unable to work for a longer period of time, but their impairment may not necessarily be terminal or expected to last at least a year.[6]

The most likely mechanism for a person with TB to qualify for DI or SSI is to have an another disabling condition, especially HIV. A diagnosis of TB in a person with HIV is considered disabling in itself according to the listing of impairments (Amendments to 20 CFR 404 *et seq.* published in 58 FR 36055, July 2, 1993). There is a separate listing for substance abuse that may also lead to disability benefits for some individuals with active TB (377).

The Role of Federal Health Insurance Programs

Although TB control falls largely to public health officials, the provision of medical services to individuals is a significant component of the

[6] For those TB patients whose disease does last at least 12 months, the SSA's listings of medical impairments do affirm that their pulmonary infections are considered disabling (377).

Figure 7-2—Hospital Admissions With a Diagnosis of Tuberculosis in 16 States[a] by Payer, 1990

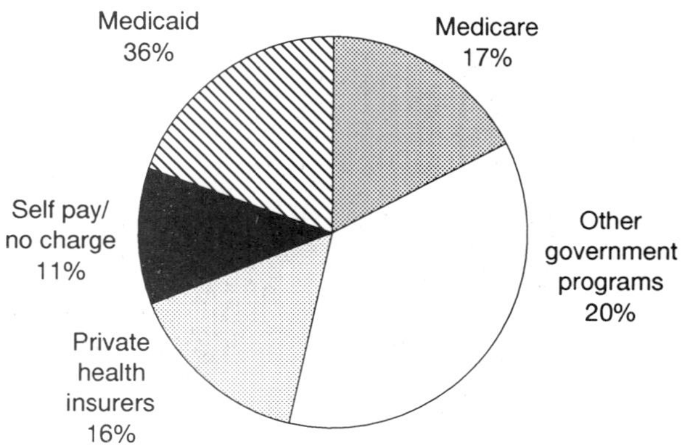

[a] States are Arizona, California, Colorado, Florida, Massachusetts, Maine, New Hampshire, New Jersey, Nevada, New York, Oregon, Pennsylvania, South Carolina, Vermont, Washington, and Wisconsin.

SOURCE: Office of Technology Assessment, 1993, based on data derived from State hospital discharge abstracts covering 100 percent of acute short-stay hospitals and U.S. Department of Veterans Affairs hospitals. Data prepared by Codman Research Group, Inc., Lebanon, New Hampshire.

overall strategy. As already described, some medical services are provided directly to patients in outpatient clinics through State and local programs that may receive some funding through grants from CDC. This medical care includes outpatient treatment of active TB and related tests and services. However, third-party insurance programs, including the Medicare and Medicaid programs that operate with Federal funds, also pay for some medical services for TB patients covered by them. As suggested in chapter 6, the role of private physicians in treating TB became more important over the 1970s and 1980s as public health programs lost their funding.

Little, if any, systematic research has been done on the role of health insurance in financing care for TB patients. However, indirect evidence suggests a significant Federal role, especially through Medicaid. A 1990 breakdown of all hospital admissions with tuberculosis as a diagnosis, in 16 States, according to payer (figure 7-2) shows that Medicaid was the single most likely payer (36 percent) with private health insurance paying for just 16 percent of admissions.[7] In total, government pays for almost three-quarters of TB hospitalizations in these States. Although not representative of the entire country, the States examined do include several with the highest burdens of tuberculosis, notably New York and California (see chapter 3). Figure 7-3 shows that in New York State, Medicaid actually pays for a majority of TB hospitalizations (57 percent). Given that being poor and lacking access to regular health care are risk factors for TB (see chapter 3), the prominence of Medicaid, a program for low-income individuals and families, is not surprising.

What types of TB patients and services are covered under Medicare and Medicaid, the two major insurance programs with Federal funding? The remainder of this chapter addresses this question.[8]

MEDICAID[9]

Medicaid is funded jointly by the Federal and State governments and administered at the State level. By Federal mandate, it provides health insurance to certain groups of low-income individuals and families including all aged, blind, and disabled recipients of SSI, mothers and children

[7] As a comparison, for hospitalizations for all diagnoses nationwide in 1991, Medicaid was the expected payer only 13 percent of the time with private health insurance covering 38 percent of admissions. These data are from the 1991 National Hospital Discharge Survey (175).

[8] The Federal Government also provides direct care to qualified veterans and active military personnel in its own health care facilities as well as health insurance to civilian dependents of active military personnel through the Civilian Health and Medical Program of the Uniformed Services program. These programs may provide or pay for its beneficiaries with tuberculosis, although Medicare and Medicaid represent the major Federal contribution in health services reimbursement.

[9] While this report was in its final publishing stages, Congress adopted legislation giving States the option to use Medicaid funds to pay for TB services only for low-income individuals with either tuberculous infection or active disease who do not otherwise qualify for Medicaid (Public Law 103-66).

who receive Aid to Families with Dependent Children (AFDC), and other categories of poor women and children. States also have the option of covering "medically needy" individuals whose high medical bills, in effect, make them poor or almost poor.

The Federal Government also requires that all categorically-eligible Medicaid beneficiaries (AFDC and SSI recipients) and some medically needy beneficiaries receive a minimum set of benefits that would cover inpatient, outpatient, laboratory, and other services. States are required to assure the availability of transportation to and from medical services and have the option of adding a variety of supplemental services to the minimum package. States receive matching Federal funds for the optional coverage they decide to provide as part of Medicaid (284,329).

While almost all inpatient, short-stay care associated with TB for Medicaid-eligible individuals would qualify for Medicaid reimbursement, concern over the eligibility of some long-term care and outpatient facilities providing TB services and a desire for flexibility in reimbursing various types of DOT has led the Health Care Financing Administration (HCFA), the Federal agency charged with administering the Federal Government's regulation of Medicaid, to issue three pieces of correspondence to help guide the States (389).

In July 1992, New York State filed an amendment to their "State Medicaid plan" explicitly discussing the funding of DOT for Medicaid-eligible patients, the only State to have made such a change to its Medicaid program. The amendment establishes three reimbursement rates for DOT services designed to give flexibility in the provision and supervision of TB treatment; the reimbursement rate depends on the setting that care is provided and the amount of effort necessary to ensure completion of treatment. Reimbursement can include the cost of food vouchers, transportation tokens, and other incentives given

Figure 7-3—New York State Hospital Admissions With a Diagnosis of Tuberculosis, by Payer, 1990

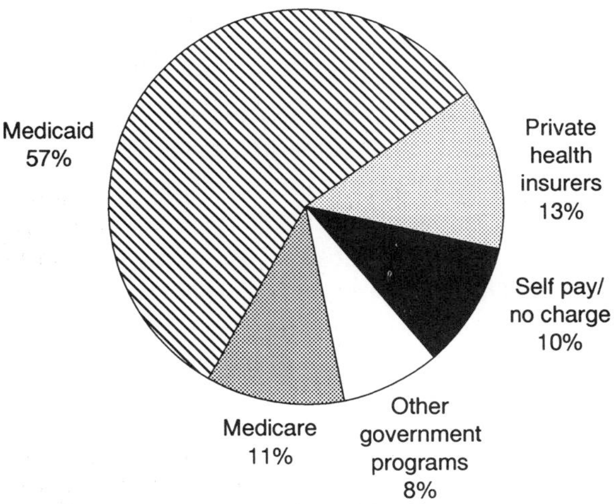

SOURCE: Office of Technology Assessment, 1993, based on data derived from state hospital discharge abstracts covering 100 percent of acute short-stay hospitals and U.S. Department of Veterans Affairs hospitals. Data prepared by Codman Research Group, Inc., Lebanon, New Hampshire.

by health care providers to encourage compliance (168,282,283,284). As of April 1993, 22 health care institutions in New York City have agreed to provide Medicaid-reimbursed DOT with a total enrollment of approximately 250 patients. The State expects the first year of the program to cost Medicaid $5.8 million in combined State and Federal funds (284,390).

HCFA estimates that $75 million in Medicaid funds went for the care of patients with tuberculosis in 1991. This estimate comprises $45 million in Federal funds and $30 million in State funds (391).

MEDICARE

Medicare provides health insurance to individuals over age 65 who have had the appropriate taxes deducted from their paychecks during their careers and to individuals who have received DI disability benefits for at least 24 months (see section on disability).[10] Both HIV, which can lead

[10] Medicare also covers individuals receiving dialysis treatment for end-stage renal disease.

to disability, and old age are also risk factors for TB as discussed in chapter 3. HCFA estimates that in 1991, $65 million in Medicare funds went for the treatment of TB (391).

Medicare consists of two types of insurance coverage. Part A covers short-term hospital stays after patients pay a deductible for each hospitalization. Hospitals are reimbursed under the diagnosis related group (DRG) system with a set amount for each hospital stay regardless of length. The actual reimbursement is based on the average historical cost of treating all patients with the same primary diagnosis. Part B covers outpatient services provided under a doctor's supervision in an office or ambulatory clinic in return for a monthly premium. Patients also pay an annual deductible and 20 percent of allowable charges.[11] Allowable charges are set by the Federal government.

For TB patients covered by Medicare, inpatient services provided in short-stay hospital and ambulatory services provided in an office or clinic under a doctor's supervision (most care provided while diagnosing active TB and treating it during its most acute phases) are almost all likely to be reimbursable. Most uncertainties about coverage center around DOT and the provision of care in specialized facilities. Although Medicare does contain some limited home health care benefits, the provision of DOT in the home would not be among them.[12] Similarly, Medicare pays for limited long-term care and skilled nursing services in certain types of federally approved facilities. To date, neither HCFA nor its regional contractors, usually private insurance companies that actually administer Medicare for the Federal Government, have undertaken any special efforts concerning Medicare coverage of TB services (389).

[11] A majority of elderly Medicare beneficiaries carry private health insurance designed to provide benefits not covered under Medicare and to help pay Medicare's deductibles and copayments (5).

[12] A recent Office of Technology Assessment report provides much more detail about current Medicare home health benefits (U.S. Congress, OTA, *Home Drug Infusion Therapy Under Medicare*, OTA-H-509, Washington, DC: U.S. Government Printing Office, May 1992).

Appendix A: Acknowledgments

OTA wishes to thank *The Continuing Challenge of Tuberculosis* workshop participants, contractors, and the individuals and organizations listed below for their assistance over the course of this study. These individuals and organizations do not necessarily approve, disapprove, or endorse this report. OTA assumes full responsibility for the report and the accuracy of its content.

Margaret Anderson
Professional Affairs
American Public Health Association
Washington, DC

Bascom Anthony
Division of Bacterial Products
Food and Drug Administration
U.S. Department of Health and Human Services
Rockville, MD

John Bass, Jr.
Division of Pulmonary and Critical Care Medicine
College of Medicine
University of South Alabama
Mobile, AL

Erin Y. Bellin
Infectious Disease Service
Montefiore Medical Center
New York, NY

Phil Bierbaum
National Institute for Occupational Safety and Health
Centers for Disease Control and Prevention
U.S. Department of Health and Human Services
Cincinnati, OH

Joel A. Block
Department of Internal Medicine
Rush-Presbyterian-St. Luke's Medical Center
Rush University
Chicago, IL

Elizabeth Bolyard
Hospital Infections Program
National Center for Infectious Diseases
Centers for Disease Control and Prevention
U.S. Department of Health and Human Services
Atlanta, GA

Lynn Bosco
Agency for Health Care Policy and Research
U.S. Department of Health and Human Services
Rockville, MD

Carmine Bozzi
Division of Tuberculosis Elimination
National Center for Prevention Services
Centers for Disease Control and Prevention
U.S. Department of Health and Human Services
Atlanta, GA

Michael J. Brennan
Laboratory of Mycobacteria
Food and Drug Administration
U.S. Department of Health and Human Services
Rockville, MD

Don Brown
Division of Tuberculosis Elimination
National Center for Prevention Services
Centers for Disease Control and Prevention
U.S. Department of Health and Human Services
Atlanta, GA

Ruth Brown
Medical Technology Assessment and Policy Research Center
Battelle
Washington, DC

Jacalyn Bryan
Governmental Affairs Committee
Association for Practitioners in Infection Control
Fairfax Station, VA

Janice E. Burr
Tuberculosis Control
Dade County Department of Health
Miami, FL

Linda A. Chiarello
Infection Control and Occupational Health Unit, AIDS Institute
Department of Health
State of New York
Albany, NY

Codman Research Group, Inc.
Lebanon, NH

Mitchell Cohen
National Center for Infectious Diseases
Centers for Disease Control and Prevention
U.S. Department of Health and Human Services
Atlanta, GA

David Cohn
Disease Control Services
Denver Department of Health and Hospitals
Denver, CO

Frank Collins
Office of Vaccine Research and Review
Food and Drug Administration
U.S. Department of Health and Human Services
Rockville, MD

George W. Comstock
Department of Epidemiology
School of Hygiene & Public Health
Johns Hopkins University
Baltimore, MD

Arthur Dannenberg, Jr.
Division of Occupational Health
School of Hygiene and Public Health
Johns Hopkins University
Baltimore, MD

Thomas Daniel
Center for International Health
School of Medicine
Case Western Reserve University
Cleveland, OH

Katherine DeVinny
Division of Clinical Research
National Institute on Drug Abuse
National Institutes of Health
U.S. Department of Health and Human Services
Rockville, MD

George DiFerdinando, Jr.
Tuberculosis Control and Refugee Health Programs
Department of Health
State of New York
Albany, NY

Samuel Dooley
Division of Tuberculosis Elimination
National Center for Prevention Services
Centers for Disease Control and Prevention
U.S. Department of Health and Human Services
Atlanta, GA

Fran Du Melle
American Lung Association
Washington, DC

Barry Eigen
Office of Disability
Social Security Administration
U.S. Department of Health and Human Services
Baltimore, MD

John Foulds
Tuberculosis Program
National Institutes of Health
U.S. Department of Health and Human Services
Bethesda, MD

Thomas R. Frieden
Bureau of Tuberculosis Control
Department of Health
City of New York
New York, NY

Jeffrey Glassroth
School of Medicine
Northwestern University
Chicago, IL

Marian Goble
National Jewish Center for Immunology and Respiratory Medicine
Denver, CO

Mark J. Goldberger
Division of Antiviral Drug Products
Food and Drug Administration
U.S. Department of Health and Human Services
Rockville, MD

Sharon Hansen
Food and Drug Administration
U.S. Department of Health and Human Services
Rockville, MD

Robert C. Hastings
Hansen's Disease Center
Louisiana State University
Baton Rouge, LA

Alan Hinman
Division of Tuberculosis Elimination
National Center for Prevention Services
Centers for Disease Control and Prevention
U.S. Department of Health and Human Services
Atlanta, GA

Philip Hopewell
Chest Service
San Francisco General Hospital
San Francisco, CA

Robert L. Hotchkiss
Tuberculosis Program
Mississippi Department of Health
Jackson, MS

Michael Iseman
Clinical Mycobacteriology Service
National Jewish Center for Immunology and Respiratory Medicine
Denver, CO

Robert R. Jacobson
Hansen's Disease Center
U.S. Department of Health and Human Services
Carville, LA

Patrick Johannes
Indian Health Service
Health Resources Services Administration
U.S. Department of Health and Human Services
Albuquerque, NM

Margarite Johnson
Robert Wood Johnson Foundation
Princeton, NJ

William Jordan, Jr.
National Vaccine Program
U.S. Department of Health and Human Services
Rockville, MD

Ruth Kasloff
Special Projects
Communications Department
American Lung Association
New York, NY

Jim Kelly
Infection Control and Employee Health
Siskin Hospital
Chattanooga, TN

Ruth Kirschstein
National Institute of General Medicine
National Institutes of Medicine
U.S. Department of Health and Human Services
Bethesda, MD

Susan J. Klein
Division of Epidemiology
Department of Health
State of New York
Albany, NY

Arata Kochi
Tuberculosis Programme
World Health Organization
Geneva, Switzerland

John Kuharik
Tuberculosis Program
Chicago Department of Health
Chicago, IL

June Lunney
Acute and Chronic Illness Branch
National Center for Nursing Research
National Institutes of Health
U.S. Department of Health and Human Services
Bethesda, MD

Jerry M. Mallick
Museum Specialist
Photographic Archives
National Gallery of Art
Washington, DC

Diane Maple
Media Relations
American Lung Association
Washington, DC

Linda McDonald
Association for Practitioners in Infection Control
Fairfax Station, VA

Jeffrey Mecaskey
Program in Tropical Disease Research
Edna McConnell Clark Foundation
New York, NY

Bess Miller
Division of Tuberculosis Elimination
National Center for Prevention Services
Centers for Disease Control and Prevention
U.S. Department of Health and Human Services
Atlanta, GA

Dennis Mitchison
Department of Bacteriology
Royal Postgraduate Medical School
London, England

Robert Moran
National AIDS Program Office
U.S. Department of Health and Human Services
Washington, DC

Sheldon Morris
Food and Drug Administration
U.S. Department of Health and Human Services
Rockville, MD

Ed Nardell
State Laboratory Institute
Massachusetts Department of Public Health
Jamaica Plain, MA

Charles Nolan
Tuberculosis Control Program
Seattle-King County Department of Public Health
Seattle, WA

Richard O'Brien
Tuberculosis Programme
World Health Organization
Geneva, Switzerland

Cynthia Palmer
Medical Technology Assessment and Policy Research Center
Battelle
Washington, DC

Mary Pendergast
Office of the Commissioner
Food and Drug Administration
U.S. Department of Health and Human Services
Rockville, MD

Gina Pugliese
Infection Control and Environmental Safety
American Hospital Association
Chicago, IL

Lynn Richmond
Montefiore Rikers Island Health Services
Montefiore Medical Center
The University Hospital for the Albert Einstein College of Medicine
New York, NY

William Rom
Department of Medicine
Division of Pulmonary and Critical Care Medicine
New York University Medical Center
New York, NY

Gary A. Roselle
Infectious Diseases
Medical Service-Central Office
U.S. Department of Veteran Affairs
Cincinnati, OH

Zeda Rosenberg
Office of the Director
National Institute of Allergy and Infectious Diseases
National Institutes of Health
U.S. Department of Health and Human Services
Bethesda, MD

John Sbarbaro
Division of General Internal Medicine
Health Sciences Center
University of Colorado
Denver, CO

John Seggerson
Division of Tuberculosis Elimination
National Center for Prevention Services
Centers for Disease Control and Prevention
U.S. Department of Health and Human Services
Atlanta, GA

Teresa Seitz
Division of Surveillance
National Institute for Occupational Safety and Health
Centers for Disease Control and Prevention
U.S. Department of Health and Human Services
Cincinnati, OH

Stephen Shaw
Health Care Financing Administration
U.S. Department of Health and Human Services
New York, NY

John Siegfried
Medical Affairs
Pharmaceutical Manufacturers Association
Washington, DC

Elaine Sloand
Office of the Director
National Heart Lung, and Blood Institute
National Institutes of Health
U.S. Department of Health and Human Services
Bethesda, MD

Peter Small
Howard Hughes Medical Institute
Stanford, CA

Dixie E. Snider, Jr.
Division of Tuberculosis Elimination
National Center for Prevention Services
Centers for Disease Control and Prevention
U.S. Department of Health and Human Services
Atlanta, GA

William Stead
Tuberculosis Program
Arkansas Department of Public Health
Little Rock, AR

Ellen Stover
Office on AIDS
National Institute of Mental Health
National Institutes of Health
U.S. Department of Health and Human Services
Rockville, MD

Esther Sumartojo
Division of Tuberculosis Elimination
National Center for Prevention Services
Centers for Disease Control and Prevention
U.S. Department of Health and Human Services
Atlanta, GA

Bruce Tempest
Internal Medicine
Gallup Indian Medical Center
Indian Health Service
Health Resources and Services Administration
U.S. Department of Health and Human Services
Gallup, NM

Kim Marie Thorburn
American Correctional Health Service Association
Honolulu, HI

Alan I. Trachtenberg
Science Policy and Analysis Branch
National Institute on Drug Abuse
National Institutes of Health
U.S. Department of Health and Human Services
Rockville, MD

Laurel Wiegand
Department of Medicine, Pulmonary Care and Critical Care Medicine
College of Medicine
Penn State University
Hershey, PA

Diana Weil
Tuberculosis Programme
World Health Organization
Geneva, Switzerland

Rebecca M. Wurtz
Department of Epidemiology
Cook County Hospital
Chicago, IL

Gerald Zelinger
Medicaid Bureau
Health Care Financing Administration
U.S. Department of Health and Human Services
Baltimore, MD

Appendix B: Abbreviations and Glossary

Abbreviations

ACET Advisory Council for the Elimination of Tuberculosis
AFB acid-fast bacilli
AFDC Aid to Families with Dependent Children program
AHCPR Agency for Health Care Policy and Research (PHS)
AI/AN American Indian or Alaskan Native
AIDS acquired immunodeficiency syndrome
ALA American Lung Association
BCG bacillus Calmette-Guérin (vaccine)
BMRC British Medical Research Council
BPHC Bureau of Primary Health Care (HRSA)
CDC Centers for Disease Control and Prevention (PHS)
CMI cell-mediated immunity
DI Disability Insurance Program (SSA)
DNA deoxyribonucleic acid
DRG Diagnosis Related Group system
DTH delayed-type hypersensitivity
DOT directly observed therapy
EMB ethambutol
FDA Food and Drug Administration (PHS)
GAO General Accounting Office (U.S. Congress)
HEPA high efficiency particulator air (filter)
HCFA Health Care Financing Administration (U.S. DHHS)
HCWs health care workers
HIV human immunodeficiency virus
HRSA Health Resources and Services Administration (PHS)
IHS Indian Health Service (PHS)
INH isoniazid
INS Immigration and Naturalization Service (U.S. Department of Justice)
IPT isoniazid preventive therapy
IUATLD International Union Against Tuberculosis and Other Lung Diseases
IVDUs intravenous drug users
M.avium ***Mycobacterium avium***
M.bovis ***Mycobacterium bovis***
MDR-TB multidrug-resistant tuberculosis
M.tb. ***Mycobacterium tuberculosis***
NCNR National Center for Nursing Research (NIH)
NCRR National Center for Research Resources (NIH)
NHLBI National Heart, Lung, and Blood Institute (NIH)
NIAID National Institute of Allergy and Infectious Diseases (NIH)
NIDA National Institute on Drug Abuse (NIH)
NIGMS National Institute of General Medical Sciences (NIH)
NIH National Institutes of Health (PHS)
NIMH National Institute of Mental Health (NIH)
NIOSH National Institute for Occupational Safety and Health (CDC)
NVPO National Vaccine Program Office (U.S. DHHS)
OSHA Occupational Health and Safety Administration (U.S. Department of Labor)
OTA Office of Technology Assessment (U.S. Congress)

PAPRs	powered air purification respirators
PAS	para-amino salicyclic acid
PCR	polymerase chain reaction
PHS	Public Health Service (U.S. DHHS)
PPD	purified protein derivative
PZA	pyrazinamide
R&D	research and development
RIF	rifampin
RVCT	"Report of a Verified Case of Tuberculosis" surveillance system (CDC)
SAMHSA	Substance Abuse and Mental Health Services Administration (PHS)
SM	streptomycin
SSA	Social Security Administration (U.S. DHHS)
SSI	Supplemental Security Income Program (SSA)
TB	tuberculosis
U.S. AID	Agency for International Development (U.S. International Development Cooperation Agency)
U.S. DHHS	U.S. Department of Health and Human Services
U.S. DVA	U.S. Department of Veterans Affairs
UV	ultraviolet light
UV-B	ultraviolet-B light
UV-C	ultraviolet-C light
WHO	World Health Organization

Terms

Acid-fast bacilli: Organisms that retain certain stains even after being washed with acid alcohol. Most are mycobacteria. When seen on a stained smear of sputum or other clinical specimen, a diagnosis of tuberculosis should be considered.

Acquired resistance: This term refers to the human-made condition of patients who are unresponsive to one or more of the primary drugs used to treat TB as a result of prior inadequate or erratic treatment. In the CDC's classification of drug resistance, this is referred to as secondary resistance. *Compare* Primary resistance, Multidrug-resistant tuberculosis, Secondary resistance, Transmitted resistance.

Active tuberculosis: The latter of the two general stages in the progression of TB. Individuals with active TB can be symptomatic and contagious—particularly if they are untreated or inadequately treated. Active TB can affect many organs or tissues; the lungs, however, are the most common site of infection. The disease can be transmitted during the active stage by persons expelling airborne particles containing tubercle bacilli through coughing, singing, speaking, or sneezing. Symptoms vary with the organ or body system involved, but generally include weakness, fever, chest pain, coughing, and when a small blood vessel is eroded, bloody sputum. *See* Tubercle bacillus, Tuberculosis.

Aid to Families with Dependent Children program: A program, established by the Social Security Act of 1935, providing cash payments to needy children (and their caretakers) who lack support because at least one parent is dead, disabled, continually absent from the home, or unemployed. Eligible families must meet income and resource criteria specified by the relevant State.

AIDS (acquired immunodeficiency syndrome): A disease caused by HIV and characterized by a deficiency of the immune system. The primary defect in AIDS is an acquired, persistent, quantitative functional depression within the T4 subset of lymphocytes. This depression often leads to infections caused by microorganisms that usually do not produce infections in individuals with normal immunity. HIV infection can be transmitted from one infected individual to another by means that include the sharing of a contaminated intravenous needle and engaging in unprotected sexual intercourse (i.e., intercourse without the use of condoms).

Alveoli: Terminal air sacs in the lung.

Anergy: The inability to mount an immune response to one or several skin-test antigens as a result of immunosuppression due to disease (e.g., HIV) or immunosuppressive drugs. Anergic individuals infected with the TB bacilli may falsely test negative with the PPD skin test.

Antimicrobial drug: Pharmaceutical agent used to kill or inhibit the growth of microorganisms in humans. *See* First-line drugs, Second-line drugs.

Attenuated live vaccine: A preparation of weakened bacteria or viruses, fractions thereof, or synthesized antigens identical or similar to those found in the disease-causing organisms, that is administered to produce or increase immunity to a particular disease. In this report, attenuated live vaccine is used in reference to BCG vaccine.

BCG (bacillus Calmette-Guérin) vaccine: A family of related vaccines, originally derived from an attenuated strain of *M.bovis*, believed to enhance the human immune system's response to infection and prevent the multiplication and dissemination of bacilli to various parts of the body. The efficacy of vaccine is still under debate. CDC recommends its use in the United States be restricted to selected high-risk populations among children.

Case rate: This term refers to the number of cases of active TB diagnosed in a given year per 100,000 population.

Caseous necrosis: The characteristic lesion of TB, it appears grossly as gray-white areas that resemble cheese.

Cavitation: The formation of hollow spaces (cavities) in the lungs.

CD4 cells: *See* T-lymphocytes.

Centers for Disease Control and Prevention: The Federal agency, established in 1973 within the Public Service of then U.S. Department of Health, Education, and Welfare (now U.S. Department of Health and Human Services), charged with the primarily responsibility for providing funding and other resources, leadership, and coordination to the Nation's tuberculosis control and prevention efforts. Prior to 1973, CDC existed as the Communicable Disease Centers.

Compliance: Refers to the completion by patients of all aspects of the treatment regimen as prescribed by the medical provider. Other terms, such as "adherence," are sometimes used.

Contact tracing: The procedure of tracing persons who have been in contact with a patient suffering from tuberculosis or other infectious diseases, with the object of discovering the source of infection and preventing its spread.

Delayed-type hypersensitivity: An immune process that occurs in response to tuberculous infection that destroys bacilli-laden unactivated macrophages. An overabundance of DTH causes most of the tissue damage characteristic of pulmonary tuberculosis.

Diagnosis: Identification of a disease or condition by a scientific evaluation of a patient's physical signs, symptoms, medical history, laboratory tests, and procedures.

Directly observed treatment: A compliance-enhancing strategy in which each dose of medication is observed by a healthcare worker or other responsible person. In this report, also referred to as directly observed therapy.

Disability: In this report, disability refers to the condition that qualifies certain patients with TB for benefits administered by programs of the U.S. Social Security Administration. The agency defines disability as an inability to engage in any substantial gainful activity by reason of any physical or mental impairment which can be expected to result in death or which has lasted or can be expected to last for a continuous period of not less than 12 months.

Disability Insurance program: *See* Social Security Disability Insurance program.

Disposable particulate respirator: A face mask that is designed to fit snugly and to filter out particles under the supervision of a health care worker or other responsible person.

Droplet nuclei: Microscopic particles (1 to 5 microns in diameter) produced by coughing, sneezing, or talking that carry tubercle bacilli and remain airborne by normal air currents in a room.

Drug-resistant tuberculosis: Tuberculosis caused by tubercle bacilli that have mutated to render them unresponsive to anti-TB drugs. *Compare* Acquired resistance, Multidrug-resistant tuberculosis, Primary resistance, Secondary resistance, and Transmitted resistance.

Drug-susceptible tuberculosis: Tuberculosis caused by tubercle bacilli that are sensitive to anti-TB drugs.

Efficacy: The probability of benefit to individuals in a defined population from a health care technology applied for a given health problem under ideal conditions.

Epidemiology: The scientific study of the distribution and occurrence of human diseases and health conditions, and their determinants.

Extrapulmonary tuberculosis: Tuberculosis in any part of the body other than the lungs. See laryngeal TB, miliary TB, osteotuberculosis, and TB meningitis.

First-line drugs: The five primary drugs—isoniazid, rifampin, pyrazinamide, ethambutol, and streptomycin—used to treat tuberculosis. Current treatment regimens for uncomplicated cases usually involves taking these drugs in two phases. *Compare* Second-line drugs.

Glucocorticoid drug: Pharmaceutical agent used to suppress the immune system to treat allergic or inflammatory diseases.

Granuloma: A nodular inflammatory lesion usually small or granular, firm, persistent, and containing compact grouped large white blood cells that ingest microbes.

HEPA (high efficiency particulate air) filter: Specialized filter that is capable of removing nearly all particles greater than 0.3 microns in diameter. May be of assistance in environmental control of tuberculosis transmission. Requires expertise in installation and maintenance.

Hepatitis: Diseases characterized primarily by inflammation of the liver. In this report, it refers to the most serious adverse effect of isoniazid, one of the drugs commonly used to treat tuberculosis.

High-risk populations: Certain demographic groups who are at a greater risk than the general U.S. public to contract a particular disease. In the case of TB, these groups include individuals who are economically disadvantaged; co-infected with HIV; foreign born; members of a racial or ethnic minority group; substance abusers; homeless; migrant farm workers; incarcerated; very young or advanced in age.

Histological: Pertaining to the study of anatomy that deals with the minute structure, composition, and function of the tissues; also called microscopical anatomy.

HIV (human immunodeficiency virus): The pathogen that causes AIDS.

HIV-seronegative: Refers to individuals who produce a negative reaction to tests that detect HIV antibodies as an indicator of HIV infection.

HIV-seropositive: Refers to individuals who produce a positive reaction to HIV antibody tests showing antibodies to HIV indicating infection with HIV.

Immunocompetent: Individuals that are capable of producing normal or adequate immune responses.

Immunocompromised: A term used to describe individuals who have a diminished or impaired immune response as a result of diseases (such as cancer or AIDS), malnutrition, or prior medical treatment involving immunosuppressive drugs or irradiation.

Immunodeficiency: A deficiency of immune response or a disorder characterized by deficiency of immune response; classified as antibody (B cell), cellular (T cell), combined deficiency, or pagocytic dysfunction disorders. Cellular immunodeficiencies are marked by recurrent infections with low-grade or opportunistic pathogens, by graft-versus-host reactions following blood transfusions, and by severe disease following immunization with live vaccines.

Immunosuppression: Refers to the suppression of natural human immune responses by infection as caused by disease, malnutrition, or prior medical treatment involving drugs or irradiation.

Immunosuppressive drugs: Pharmaceutical agents that suppress natural human immune responses to prevent the rejection of grafts or organ transplants.

Immunotherapy: The treatment of disease by the administration to the patient of antibody raised in another individual or another species (passive immunotherapy) or by immunizing the patient with antigens appropriate to the disease (active immunotherapy).

Incidence: The frequency of new occurrences of disease within a defined time interval. The incidence rate is the number of new cases of specified disease divided by the number of people in a population over a specified period of time, usually 1 year.

Incident cases: New cases of a disease within a defined time interval.

INH (isoniazid) preventive therapy: The treatment of tuberculous infection with the antibacterial drug isoniazid to prevent progression of tuberculous infection to active disease.

Laryngeal tuberculosis: Tuberculosis of the larynx.

Latent tuberculosis: *See* Tuberculous infection.

Lesion: Any abnormal discontinuity of tissue or loss of function. A wound, injury, or one of the individual points or patches of a multifocal disease.

Liquefaction: A disease-related process of solid tissues decomposing into liquid.

Lymphadenitis: *See* Tuberculous lymphadenitis.

Macrophage: A large and versatile immune cell found in many tissues of the body that has an important role in host defense mechanisms by ingesting microbes, including bacteria, viruses, fungi, and other foreign particles.

Medicaid: A government medical assistance program that pays for medical expenses for the poor and certain other classes of uninsured people, established by the Title XIX of the Social Security Act of 1965. Each State administers its own program. Medicaid is funded by both the State and Federal Governments.

Medicare: A federally administered health insurance program covering the cost of services for people 65 years of age or older, receiving Social Security Disability Insurance payments for at least 2 years, or with end-stage renal disease. Medicare consists of two separate but coordinated programs—hospital insurance (Part A) and supplementary medical insurance (Part B). Health insurance protection is available to qualified persons without regard to income.

Meningitis: *See* Tuberculosis meningitis.

Miliary tuberculosis: Tuberculosis of various body organs and tissues resulting from millet-like (miliary) lesions or life-threatening meningitis that have been transported through the bloodstream from the initial site of infection (usually the lungs). *See* Active TB, Latent TB, *Mycobacterium TB*, Tubercle bacillus, Tuberculosis, Tuberculous infection.

Multidrug-resistant tuberculosis: Tuberculosis that occurs in persons who are unresponsive to two or more of the anti-TB drugs used to treat the disease, particularly the two most powerful ones—isoniazid and rifampin. *See* Acquired resistance, Primary resistance, Transmitted resistance.

Mycobacterium: The name of the bacterial family that causes TB and other infectious diseases in humans and animals. In this report, only three members of this category are discussed—*Mycobacterium avium*, *Mycobacterium bovis*, and *Mycobacterium tuberculosis*.

Mycobacterium avium: A non-tuberculous mycobacterial infection that occurs frequently in individuals with AIDS and can lead to serious complications and death.

Mycobacterium tuberculosis: The bacteria that causes tuberculosis in humans. *See Mycobacterium*, Tuberculosis.

National Action Plan to Combat MDR-TB: In 1992, following the recent worsening of the TB problem as indicated by the series of MDR-TB outbreaks, a national plan was released by CDC to enhance the Federal Government's 1988 strategic plan, "National Action Plan to Combat Multidrug-Resistant Tuberculosis." The Action Plan identified a detailed plan to control drug-susceptible TB and MDR-TB implementation involving an array of Government agencies and professional organizations. See box 7-B for a summary of key points of the Action Plan.

Orphan drug: A drug product discovered and developed for the treatment of a rare disease or a drug product not expected to produce enough revenue to cover its R&D or manufacturing and distribution costs.

Osteotuberculosis: Tuberculosis of the bone.

Polymerase chain reaction: A laboratory process through which repeated cycling of the reaction reproduces a specific region of DNA, yielding millions of copies from the original. The process has been adapted for the rapid detection of TB, although such tests remain expensive and require significant expertise to use.

Powered air purification respirators: Powered, halfmask respirators equipped with high-efficiency particulate filters that are specialized filters capable of removing nearly all particles from the air. These devices have been used as environmental control measure by health care workers to control the transmission of TB.

Prevalence: In epidemiology, the number of cases of diseases, infected persons, or persons with disabilities or some other condition, present at a particular time and in relation to the size of the population. Also called "prevalence rate." *Compare* Incidence.

Prevalent cases: Total number of cases of a disease present in a defined population at a particular time.

Prevention: The averting of disease, traditionally characterized as primary, secondary, and tertiary prevention. Primary prevention aims at avoiding disease altogether. Secondary prevention strategies detect disease in its early stages of development, with the hope of improving outcome. Tertiary prevention attempts to arrest further deterioration in individuals who already suffer from a disease.

Primary resistance: This term refers to a naturally occurring biological phenomenon in patients who are unresponsive to the common drugs used to treat the tuberculosis but are not known to have received prior treatment. Also called transmitted resistance in this report. In CDC's classification, primary resistance also refers to infection by a TB organism already drug resistant. *Compare* Acquired resistance, Multidrug-resistant tuberculosis, Secondary resistance, Transmitted resistance.

Pulmonary tuberculosis: Tuberculosis of the lungs, the most common form of the disease.

Report of a Verified Case of Tuberculosis: The individual TB case report sent by State and local health authorities to CDC that allows uniform collection and analysis of data on TB cases in the United States.

Research and development: In this report, research and development refers to Federal funding of the activities to detect, prevent, and control the TB problem in the United States, including basic scientific inquiry, behavioral research, health services research, development of new or improved diagnostic tools, infection control, and clinical research into vaccines and treatment.

Resistance: *See* Drug-resistant tuberculosis.

Second-line drugs: Drugs used to treat TB when a patient is unresponsive to treatment with first-line drugs. The second-line drugs include amikacin, capreomycin, cycloserine, ethionamide, kanamycin, and p-aminosalicyclic acid. *Compare* First-line drugs.

Secondary resistance: *See* Acquired resistance.

Sensitivity: One measure of the validity (or accuracy) of a diagnostic or screening test: the percentage of all those who actually have the condition being tested who are correctly identified as positive by the test. Operationally, it is the number of true positive test results divided by the number of patients that actually have the disease (true positives divided by the sum of true positives plus false negatives). *Compare* Specificity.

Social Security Disability Insurance program: A Federal social insurance program for workers who have contributed to the social security retirement program and become disabled before retirement age. Beneficiaries receive monthly cash payments.

Specificity: One measure of the validity (or accuracy) of a diagnostic or screening test: the percentage of all those who do not have the condition being tested who are correctly identified as negative by the test. Operationally, it is the number of true test negatives (all those with a negative test result who actually do not have the condition being tested for) divided by the sum of true negatives plus false positives (i.e., all those who do not have the condition). *Compare* Sensitivity.

Sputum smear-positive: Sputum that is positive for AFB when stained and viewed under a microscope. Individuals with TB who are sputum smear-positive for AFB are considered more infectious than those with smear-negative sputum.

Supplemental Security Income: A Federal income support program for low-income disabled, aged, and blind persons. Eligibility for the monthly cash payments is based on the individual's current status without regard to previous work or contributions to a trust fund. Some States supplement the Federal benefit.

Surveillance: Constant observation of an area to determine the level of disease activity. In this report, surveillance refers to public health activities that include maintaining registries of clinical information concerning cases and suspected cases and conducting contact investigations to locate additional cases.

T-lymphocytes: Specialized white blood cells involved in the body's immune response. B-lymphocytes originate in the bone marrow and when stimulated by an antigen produce circulating antibodies (humoral immunity). T-lymphocytes are produced in the bone marrow and mature in the thymus gland and engage in a type of defense that does not depend directly on antibody attack (cell-mediated immunity).

Transmitted resistance: This term refers to TB drug resistance that occurs when a strain of TB already resistant to one or more anti-TB drugs is transmitted to a new case (e.g., in institutional settings) and results in resistance to the same number and types of drugs as in the source case. *Compare* Acquired resistance, Multidrug-resistant tuberculosis, Primary resistance, Secondary resistance.

Tubercle bacillus: A bacillus (bacteria) causing tuberculosis; usually refers to *Mycobacterium tuberculosis*, the principal cause of human tuberculosis.

Tuberculin skin test: A method for demonstrating infection with *mycobacterium tuberculosis* in which antigenic material from *M.tb.* cultures is introduced into the skin, either intradermally or percutaneously.

Tuberculosis: A treatable infectious disease caused by some species of *Mycobacteria*. Individuals can contract TB when exposed to airborne particles containing tubercle bacilli through inhalation (i.e., coughing, singing, speaking, or sneezing). TB has two general stages: tuberculous infection (latent tuberculosis) and active tuberculosis. The first stage is asymptotic and ***not*** contagious to others, whereas active TB is symptomatic and contagious—particularly if untreated or inadequately treated. *See* Active TB, Latent TB, *Mycobacterium TB*, Tubercle bacillus, Tuberculous infection. *See also* Extrapulmonary TB, Pulmonary TB, Laryngeal TB, Miliary TB, and TB meningitis.

Tuberculosis meningitis: Tuberculosis of the membranes surrounding the brain and spinal cord.

Tuberculous infection: Condition in which living tubercle bacilli are present in an individual, without producing clinically active disease. Infected individuals usually have a positive tuberculin skin test, but not symptoms related to the infection, and are not infectious. TB infection is necessary to develop active TB disease. Also known as latent tuberculosis.

Tuberculous lymphadenitis: Tuberculosis of the lymph nodes.

Ultraviolet radiation: A form of invisible electromagnetic radiation having a shorter wavelength than that of the violet end of the spectrum and longer than that of x-rays. In this report, ultraviolet radiation refers to an infection control method using ultraviolet light sources to kill bacteria. These lights can be part of ceiling or wall fixtures or found within air ducts of recirculating ventilation systems.

References

1. Addington, W.W., Albert, R.K., Bass, J.B., Jr., et al., "Non-Drug Issues Related to the Treatment of TB," *Chest* 87(2):S125-S128, 1985.
2. Alcabes, P., Vossenas, P., Cohen, R., et al., "Compliance With Isoniazid Prophylaxis in Jail," *American Review of Respiratory Disease* 140:1194-1197, 1989.
3. Aldovini, A., and Young, R.A., "Humoral and Cell-Mediated Immune Responses to Live Recombinant BCG-HIV Vaccines," *Nature* 351: 479-482, 1991.
4. Alexander, E., Chief of Litigation, American Civil Liberties Union National Prison Project, Washington, DC, personal communication, June 30, 1993.
5. American Association of Retired Persons, *Consumer Awareness of Medigap Insurance: Findings of a National Survey of Older Americans*, prepared by Market Facts, Inc. (Washington, DC: American Association of Retired Persons, 1989).
6. American Thoracic Society, "Treatment of Tuberculosis and Tuberculous Infection in Adults and Children," *American Review of Respiratory Disease* 134:355-363, 1986.
7. American Thoracic Society, "Diagnostic Standards and Classification of Tuberculosis," *American Review of Respiratory Disease* 142:725-735, 1990.
8. American Thoracic Society, "Control of Tuberculosis in the United States," *American Review of Respiratory Disease* 146:1623-1633, 1992.
9. Annas, G.J., "Control of Tuberculosis—the Law and the Public's Health," *New England Journal of Medicine* 328(8):585-588, 1993.
10. Anthony, B.F., Division of Bacterial Products, Center for Biologics Evaluation and Research, Food and Drug Administration, U.S. Department of Health and Human Service, Rockville, MD, personal communication, April 1993.
11. Armbruster, C., Junker, W., Vetter, N., et al., "Disseminated Bacilli Calmette-Guerin Infection in an AIDS Patient 30 Years After BCG Vaccination," *Journal of Infectious Diseases* 162:1216, 1990.
12. Assistant Secretary for Health's Public Health Service Task Force to Strengthen Public Health in the United States, "A Plan to Strengthen Public Health in the United States," *Public Health Reports* 106(suppl. 1):1-86, 1991.
13. Bailey, W.C., Byrd, R.B., Glassroth, J.L., et al., "Preventive Treatment of Tuberculosis: Report of the National Consensus Conference on Tuberculosis," *Chest* 87(2):128S-132S, 1985.
14. Barnes, P.F., Bloch, A.B., Davidson, P.T., et al., "Tuberculosis in Patients With Human Immunodeficiency Virus Infection," *New England Journal of Medicine* 324(23):1644-1650, 1991.
15. Barrett-Connor, E., "The Epidemiology of Tuberculosis in Physicians," *Journal of the American Medical Association* 241:33-38, 1979.
16. Barry, M.A., Wall, C., Shirley, L., et al., "Tuberculosis Screening in Boston's Homeless Shelters," *Public Health Reports* 101(5): 487-498, 1986.

17. Bass, J.B., Jr., "Tuberculin Test, Preventive Therapy, and Elimination of Tuberculosis," *American Review of Respiratory Disease* 141:812-813, 1990.
18. Bass, J.B., Jr., "The Tuberculin Skin Test," *Tuberculosis: A Comprehensive International Approach*, L.B. Reichman and E.S. Hershfield (eds.)(New York, NY: Marcel Dekker, Inc., 1993).
19. Bass, J.B., Jr., Chairman, Advisory Committee for the Elimination of Tuberculosis, Centers for Disease Control and Prevention, Public Health Service, U.S. Department of Health and Human Services, unpublished minutes, Atlanta, GA, Apr. 2-3, 1992.
20. Beck-Sague, C., Dooley, S.W., Hutton, M.D., et al., "Hospital Outbreak of Multidrug-Resistant *Mycobacterium tuberculosis* Infections: Factors in Transmission to Staff and HIV-Infected Patients," *Journal of the American Medical Association* 268(10):1280-1286, 1992.
21. Beekman, S.E., Osterholm, M.T., Henderson, D.K., "Tuberculosis in the Healthcare Setting in the 1990s: From Bird Island to the Bronx," *Infection Control and Hospital Epidemiology* 14:228-232, 1993.
22. Bell, D., Chief of AIDS Activity, Hospital Infections Program, Centers for Disease Control and Prevention, Public Health Service, U.S. Department of Health and Human Services, Atlanta, GA, personal communication, December 1992.
23. Bellin, E.Y., Fletcher, D.D., and Safyer, S.M., "Association of Tuberculosis Infection With Increased Time in or Admission to the New York City Jail System," *Journal of the American Medical Association* 269(17): 2228-2231, 1993.
24. Bierbaum, P., Chief, Division of Physical Sciences and Engineering, National Institute for Occupational Safety and Health, Centers for Disease Control and Prevention, Public Health Service, U.S. Department of Health and Human Services, Cincinnati, OH, personal communication, June 7, 1993.
25. Bloch, A.B., Medical Officer, Surveillance and Epidemiology Branch, Division of Tuberculosis Elimination, Centers for Disease Control and Prevention, Public Health Service, U.S. Department of Health and Human Services, Atlanta, GA, notes from Advisory Committee for the Elimination of Tuberculosis meeting, 1992.
26. Bloch, A.B., Medical Officer, Surveillance and Epidemiology Branch, Division of Tuberculosis Elimination, Centers for Disease Control and Prevention, Public Health Service, U.S. Department of Health and Human Services, Atlanta, GA, personal communication, December 1992.
27. Bloch, A.B., Rieder, H.L., and Kelly, G.D., "The Epidemiology of Tuberculosis in the United States," *Seminars in Respiratory Infections* 4(3):157-170, 1989.
28. Bloch, A.B., Rieder, H.L., Kelly, G.D., et al., "The Epidemiology of Tuberculosis in the United States: Implications for Diagnosis and Treatment," *Clinics in Chest Medicine* 10(3):297-313, 1989.
29. Bloom, B.R., Professor, Albert Einstein College of Medicine, Department of Microbiology and Immunology, New York, NY, personal communication, Mar. 17, 1993.
30. Bloom, B.R., Professor, Albert Einstein College of Medicine, Department of Microbiology and Immunology, New York, NY, personal communication, Mar. 23, 1993.
31. Bloom, B.R., and Murray, C.J.L., "Tuberculosis: Commentary on a Reemergent Killer," *Science* 257:1055-1064, 1992.
32. Bosco L., Medical Officer, Agency for Health Care Policy and Research, Public Health Service, U.S. Department of Health and Human Services, Rockville, MD, personal communication, June 8, 1993.
33. Boudes, P., Sobel, A., Deforges, L., et al., "Disseminated *Mycobacterium bovis* Infection From BCG Vaccination and HIV Infection," *Journal of the American Medical Association* 262:2386, 1989.
34. Boudreau, A.Y., Medical Officer, National Institute for Occupational Safety and Health, Centers for Disease Control and Prevention, Public Health Service, U.S. Department of Health and Human Services, Cincinnati, OH, personal communication, Apr. 21, 1993.

35. Bozzi, C., Assistant to the Director for Tuberculosis Control, Division of Tuberculosis Elimination, National Center for Prevention Services, Centers for Disease Control and Prevention, Public Health Service, U.S. Department of Health and Human Services, Atlanta, GA, personal communication, May 6, 1993.
36. Bozzi, C., Assistant to the Director for Tuberculosis Control, Division of Tuberculosis Elimination, National Center for Prevention Services, Centers for Disease Control and Prevention, Public Health Service, U.S. Department of Health and Human Services, Atlanta, GA, May 10, 1993; based on data from M. McDiarmid, Occupational Safety and Health Administration, U.S. Department of Labor, Washington, DC.
37. Bozzi, C., Assistant to the Director for Tuberculosis Control, Division of Tuberculosis Elimination, National Center for Prevention Services, Centers for Disease Control and Prevention, Public Health Service, U.S. Department of Health and Human Services, Atlanta, GA, personal communication, June 14, 1993.
38. Bozzi, C., Assistant to the Director for Tuberculosis Control, Division of Tuberculosis Elimination, National Center for Prevention Services, Centers for Disease Control and Prevention, Public Health Service, U.S. Department of Health and Human Services, Atlanta, GA, personal communication, July 9, 1993.
39. Braun, M.M., Cote, T.R., and Robkin, C.S., "Trends in Death With Tuberculosis During the AIDS Era," *Journal of the American Medical Association* 269(22):2865-2868, 1993.
40. Braun, M.M., Byers, R.H., Heyward, W.L., et al., "Acquired Immunodeficiency Syndrome and Extrapulmonary Tuberculosis in the United States," *Archives of Internal Medicine* 150:1913-1916, 1990.
41. Braun, M.M., Truman, B.I., Maguire, B., et al., "Increasing Incidence of Tuberculosis in a Prison Inmate Population: Association With HIV Infection," *Journal of the American Medical Association* 261:393-397, 1989.
42. Bregere, P., "BCG Vaccination and AIDS," *Bulletin of the International Union Against Tuberculosis and Lung Disease* 63:40-41, 1988.
43. Brenner, E., and Poszik, C., "Case Holding," *Tuberculosis: A Comprehensive International Approach*, L.B. Reichman and E.S. Hershfield (eds.)(New York, NY: Marcel Dekker, Inc., 1993).
44. Brisson-Noel, A., Aznar, C., Chureau, C., et al., "Diagnosis of Tuberculosis by DNA Amplification in Clinical Practice Evaluation," *Lancet* 338:364-366, 1991.
45. Brudney, K., and Dobkin, J., "Resurgent Tuberculosis in New York City: Human Immunodeficiency Virus, Homelessness, and the Decline of Tuberculosis Control Programs," *American Review of Respiratory Disease* 144:745-749, 1991.
46. Brudney, K., and Dobkin, J., "A Tale of Two Cities: Tuberculosis Control in Nicaragua and New York City," *Seminars in Respiratory Infections* 6(4):261-272, 1991.
47. Buddenberg, B., Acting Associate Commissioner for Detention and Deportation, Immigration and Naturalization Service, U.S. Department of Justice, Washington, DC, personal communication, July 2, 1993.
48. Busillo, C.P., Lessnau, K.-D., and Sanjana, V., "Multidrug Resistant *Mycobacterium tuberculosis* in Patients With Human Immunodeficiency Virus Infection," *Chest* 102:797-801, 1992.
49. Califano, J.A., Jr., "Three-Headed Dog From Hell. The Staggering Public Health Threat Posed by AIDS, Substance Abuse and Tuberculosis," *Washington Post*, December 21, 1992, p. A22.
50. Castro, K.G., and Dooley, S.W., "*Mycobacterium tuberculosis* Transmission in Healthcare Settings: Is It Influenced by Coinfection With Human Immunodeficiency Virus?" *Infection Control and Hospital Epidemiology* 14:65-66, 1993.
51. Cauthen, G.M., Kilburn, J.O., Kelly, G.D., et al., "Resistance to Antituberculous Drugs in Patients With and Without Prior Treatment: Survey of 31 State and Large City Laboratories, 1982-1986," *American Review of Respiratory Disease* 137(4)(suppl.):260, 1988.

52. Chaisson, R.E., and McAvinue, S., ''Control of Tuberculosis During Aerosol Therapy Administration,'' *Respiratory Care* 36(9):1017-1025, 1991.
53. Chaulet, P., ''Compliance With Chemotherapy for Tuberculosis. Responsibilities of the Health Ministry and of Physicians,'' *Bulletin of the International Union Against Tuberculosis and Lung Disease* 66(suppl.):33-35, 1990.
54. Chawla, P.K., Klapper, P.J., Kamholz, S.L., et al., ''Drug-Resistant Tuberculosis in an Urban Population Including Patients at Risk for Human Immunodeficiency Virus Infection,'' *American Review of Respiratory Disease* 146:280-284, 1992.
55. Cielsielski, S.D., Seed, J.R., Esposito, D.H., et al., ''The Epidemiology of Tuberculosis Among North Carolina Migrant Farm Workers,'' *Journal of the American Medical Association* 265:1715-1719, 1991.
56. City of Chicago, Department of Health, Tuberculosis Control Program, ''Tuberculosis, Morbidity and Mortality Report 1991,'' Chicago, IL, Aug. 25, 1991.
57. City of New York, Department of Health, Bureau of Tuberculosis Control, ''Tuberculosis in New York City 1991. Information Summary,'' New York, NY, 1991.
58. Clarke, A., and Rudd, P., ''Neonatal BCG Immunisation,'' *Archives of Disease in Childhood* 67:473-474, 1992.
59. Clemens, J.D., Chuong, J.J.H., and Feinstein, A.R., ''The BCG Controversy. A Methodological and Statistical Reappraisal,'' *Journal of the American Medical Association* 249(17):2362-2369, 1983.
60. Clermont, H., Johnson, M., Coberly, J., et al., ''Tolerance of Short Course TB Chemoprophylaxis in HIV-Infected Individuals,'' (Abstract No. WB 2363:273) presented at ''VII International Conference on AIDS,'' Florence, Italy, 1991.
61. Cohn, D.L., Catlin, B.J., Peterson, K.L., et al., ''A 62-Dose, 6-Month Therapy for Pulmonary and Extrapulmonary Tuberculosis. A Twice-Weekly, Directly Observed, and Cost-Effective Regimen,'' *Annals of Internal Medicine* 112 (6):407-415, 1990.
62. Combs, D.L., O'Brien, R.J., and Geiter, L.J., ''USPHS Tuberculosis Short-Course Chemotherapy Trial 21: Effectiveness, Toxicity, and Acceptability. Report of Final Results,'' *Annals of Internal Medicine* 112(6):397-406, 1990
63. Comstock, G.W., ''Identification of an Effective Vaccine Against Tuberculosis,'' *American Review of Respiratory Disease* 138:479-480, 1988.
64. Comstock, G.W., ''Prevention of Tuberculosis,'' *Bulletin of the International Union Against Tuberculosis and Lung Disease* 66(suppl.):9-11, 1990/1991.
65. Comstock, G.W., ''Prevention of Tuberculosis Among Tuberculin Reactors: Maximizing Benefits, Minimizing Risks,'' *Journal of the American Medical Association* 256(19):2729-2730, 1986.
66. Comstock, G.W., and Cauthen, G.M., ''Epidemiology of Tuberculosis,'' *Tuberculosis: A Comprehensive International Approach*, L.B. Reichman and E.S. Hershfield (eds.)(New York, NY: Marcel Dekker, Inc., 1993).
67. Cote, T.R., Nelson, M.R., Anderson, S.P., et al., ''The Present and the Future of AIDS and Tuberculosis in Illinois,'' *American Journal of Public Health* 80(8):950-953, 1990.
68. Curtis, R., Friedman, S.R., Neaigus, A., et al., ''TB Among Injecting Drug Users: Potential Negative Effects of Current Strategies,'' National Development and Research Institute, Inc., New York, NY, manuscript submitted for publication, 1993.
69. Daley, C.L., Small, P.M., Schecter, G.F., et al., ''An Outbreak of Tuberculosis With Accelerated Progression Among Persons Infected With the Human Immunodeficiency Virus: An Analysis Using Restriction-Fragment-Length Polymorphisms,'' *New England Journal of Medicine* 326(4):231-235, 1992.
70. Daniel, T.M., ''The Rapid Diagnosis of Tuberculosis: A Selective Review,'' *Journal of Laboratory Clinical Medicine* 116(3):277-282, 1990.
71. Dannenberg, A.M., Jr., Immune Mechanisms in the Pathogenesis of Pulmonary Tuberculosis,'' *Reviews of Infectious Diseases* II(suppl. 2):S369-S378, 1989.

72. Dannenberg, A.M., Jr., "Delayed-Type Hypersensitivity and Cell-Mediated Immunity in the Pathogenesis of Tuberculosis," *Immunology Today* 12(7):228-233, 1991.
73. Dannenberg, A.M., Jr., "Immunopathogenesis of Pulmonary Tuberculosis," *Hospital Practice* 28:33-40, 1993.
74. Dannenberg, A.M., Jr., and Tomashefski, J.F., Jr., "Pathogenesis of Pulmonary Tuberculosis," *Pulmonary Diseases and Disorders, 2nd Edition*, A.P. Fishman (ed.)(New York, NY: McGraw-Hill, 1988).
75. Davidson, P.T., and Le, H.Q., "Drug Treatment of Tuberculosis—1992," *Drugs* 43(5):651-673, 1992.
76. DeCock, K.M., Soro, B., Coulibaly, I.M., et al., "Tuberculosis and HIV Infection in Sub-Saharan Africa," *Journal of the American Medical Association* 268(12):1581-1587, 1992.
77. DiPerri, G., Cruciani, M., Danzi, M.C., et al., "Nosocomial Epidemic of Active Tuberculosis Among HIV-Infected Patients," *Lancet* 2:1502-1504, 1989.
78. Dooley, S.W., Division of Tuberculosis Elimination, Centers of Disease Control and Prevention, Public Health Service, U.S. Department of Health and Human Services, "Occupational Health and Safety," paper presentation at "The Dual Epidemics of TB and AIDS: Health Care Policy, Professional Practice, Law and Ethics," New York, NY, Dec. 5, 1992.
79. Dooley, S.W., National Center for Prevention Services, Centers for Disease Control and Prevention, Public Health Service, U.S. Department of Health and Human Services, Atlanta, GA, personal communication, Mar. 23, 1993.
80. Dooley, S.W., Jarvis, W.R., Martone, W.J., et al., "Multidrug-Resistant Tuberculosis," *Annals Internal of Medicine* 117(3):257-259, 1992.
81. Dooley, S.W., Villarino, M.E., Lawrence, M., et al., "Nosocomial Transmission of Tuberculosis in a Hospital Unit for HIV-Infected Patients," *Journal of the American Medical Association* 267(19):2632-2635, 1992.
82. Doster, B.D., Caras, G.J., and Snider, D.E., Jr., "A Continuing Survey of Primary Drug Resistance in Tuberculosis, 1961-1968," *American Review of Respiratory Disease* 113:419-425, 1976.
83. Dubler, N.N., Bayer, R., Landesman, S., et al., "Tuberculosis in the 1990s: Ethical, Legal, and Public Policy Issues in Screening, Treatment, and the Protection of Those in Congregate Facilities. A Report From the Working Group on TB and HIV," *The Tuberculosis Revival: Individual Rights and Societal Obligations in a Time of AIDS, Special Report* (New York, NY: United Hospital Fund of New York, 1992).
84. Dubos, R., and Dubos, J., *The White Plague: Tuberculosis, Man, and Society* (New Brunswick, NJ: Rutgers University Press, 1952; reprinted 1992).
85. DuMelle, F., Deputy Managing Director, American Lung Association, Washington, DC, personal communication, June 15, 1993.
86. East African/British Medical Research Council Study, "Results at 5 Years of a Controlled Comparison of a 6-Month and a Standard 18-Month Regimen of Chemotherapy for Pulmonary Tuberculosis," *American Review of Respiratory Disease* 115:3-8, 1977.
87. Edlin, B.R., Tokars, J.I., Grieco, M.H., et al., "An Outbreak of Multidrug-Resistant Tuberculosis Among Hospitalized Patients With the Acquired Immunodeficiency Syndrome," *New England Journal of Medicine* 326:1514-1521, 1992.
88. Eigen, B., Deputy Director, Division of Medical and Vocational Policy, Office of Disability, Social Security Administration, U.S. Department of Health and Human Services, Baltimore, MD, personal communication, June 7, 1993.
89. Eisenach, K.D., Sifford, M.D., Cave, M.D., et al., "Detection of Mycobacterium Tuberculosis in Sputum Samples Using a Polymerase Chain Reaction," *American Review of Respiratory Disease* 144:1160-1163, 1991.
90. Elovich, R., Isbell, M.T., Jacobs, S.L., et al., "Developing a System for Tuberculosis Prevention and Care in New York City," *The Tuberculosis Revival: Individual Rights and Societal Obligations in a Time of AIDS, Special Report* (New York, NY: United Hospital Fund of New York, 1992).

91. Etkind, S., ''Contact Tracing,'' State Laboratory Institute, Massachusetts Department of Public Health, Boston, MA, unpublished manuscript, 1992.
92. Etkind, S., ''Delivery of Tuberculosis Treatment,'' contract report prepared for the Office of Technology Assessment, U.S. Congress, Washington DC, May 13, 1993.
93. Etkind, S.C., ''The Role of the Public Health Department in Tuberculosis,'' State Laboratory Institute, Massachusetts Department of Public Health, Boston, MA, manuscript submitted for publication, 1993.
94. Etkind, S., Boutotte, J., Ford, J., et al., ''Treating Hard-to-Treat Tuberculosis Patients in Massachusetts,'' *Seminars in Respiratory Infections* 6(4):273-282, 1991.
95. Farmer, P., Robin, S., Ramilus, S.L., et al., ''Tuberculosis, Poverty, and 'Compliance': Lessons from Rural Haiti,'' *Seminars in Respiratory Infections* 6:254-260, 1991.
96. Fauci, A., Director, National Institute of Allergy and Infectious Disease, National Institutes of Health, Public Health Service, U.S. Department of Health and Human Services, testimony before the Subcommittee on Health and the Environment, Committee on Energy and Commerce, U.S. House of Representatives, Washington, DC, Mar. 29, 1993.
97. Ferebee, S.H., ''Controlled Chemophophylaxis Trials in Tuberculosis: A General Review,'' *Advances in Tuberculosis Research* 17:28-106, 1970.
98. Fine, P.E.M., ''The BCG Story: Lessons From the Past and Implications for the Future,'' *Review Infectious Diseases* 11(suppl. 2):S353-S359, 1989.
99. Fine, P.E.M., and Rodrigues, L.C., ''Mycobacterial Diseases,'' *Lancet* 335:1016-1020, 1990.
100. Fischl, M.A., Daikos, G.L., Uttamchandani, R.B., et al., ''Clinical Presentation and Outcome of Patients With HIV Infection and Tuberculosis Caused by Multiple-Drug-Resistant Bacilli,'' *Annals of Internal of Medicine* 117:184-190, 1992.
101. Fischl, M.A., Uttamchandani, R.B., and Daikos, G.L., ''An Outbreak of Tuberculosis Caused by Multiple-Drug-Resistant Tubercule Bacilli Among Patients With HIV Infection,'' *Annals of Internal Medicine* 117(3):177-183, 1992.
102. Fitzgerald, J.M., and Gafni, A., ''A Cost-Effectiveness Analysis of the Routine Use of Isoniazid Prophlyaxis in Patients With a Positive Mantoux Skin Test,'' *American Review of Respiratory Disease* 142:848-853, 1990.
103. FitzGerald, J.M., Grzybowski, S., and Allen, E.A., ''The Impact of Human Immunodeficiency Virus Infection on Tuberculosis and Its Control,'' *Chest* 100(1):191-200, 1991.
104. Foulds, J., Tuberculosis Program Officer, National Institute on Allergy and Infectious Diseases, National Institutes of Health, Public Health Service, U.S. Department of Health and Human Services, Rockville, MD, personal communication, February 1993.
105. Fox, W., ''Compliance of Patients and Physicians: Experience and Lesions From Tuberculosis—I,'' *British Medical Journal* 287:33-35, 1983.
106. Frampton, M.W., ''An Outbreak of Tuberculosis Among Hospital Personnel Caring for a Patient With a Skin Ulcer,'' *Annals of Internal Medicine* 117(4):312-313,1992.
107. Frieden, T.R., Sterling, T., Pablos-Mendez, A., et al., ''The Emergence of Drug-Resistant Tuberculosis in New York City,'' *New England Journal of Medicine* 328(8):521-526, 1993.
108. Frodyma, F., Acting Director of Policy, Occupational Safety and Health Administration, U.S. Department of Labor, Washington, DC, personal communication, Apr. 22, 1993.
109. Geiseler, P.J., Nelson, K.E., Crispen, R.G., et al., ''Tuberculosis in Physicians: A Continuing Problem,'' *American Review of Respiratory Disease* 133:733-778, 1986.
110. Geiter, L.J., ''Contribution of Pyrazinamide to Antituberculosis Chemotherapy,'' (letter) *Journal of Infectious Disease* 164:610, 1991.
111. Geiter, L.T., ''Preventive Therapy for Tuberculosis,'' *Tuberculosis: A Comprehensive International Approach*, L.B. Reichman and E.S. Hershfield (eds.)(New York, NY: Marcel Dekker, Inc., 1993).

112. Glaser, J.B., and Greifinger, R.B., "Correctional Health Care: A Public Health Opportunity," *Annals of Internal Medicine* 118:139-145, 1993.
113. Glassroth, J., "The Physician's Role in Tuberculosis Prevention," *Clinics in Chest Medicine* 10(3):365-374, 1989.
114. Glassroth, J., Tuberculosis Treatment: Risk, Benefit, and Perspective," *Chest* 99(2):266-267, 1991.
115. Glassroth, J., Bailey, W.C., Hopewell, P.C., et al., "Why Tuberculosis Is Not Prevented," *American Review of Respiratory Disease* 141:1236-1240, 1990.
116. Goble, M., "Drug-Resistant Tuberculosis," *Seminars in Respiratory Infections* 1(4):220-229, 1986.
117. Goble, M., Staff Physician, National Jewish Center for Immunology and Respiratory Medicine, Denver, CO, personal communication, June 1993.
118. Goble, M., Iseman, M.D., Madsen, L.A., et al., "Treatment of 171 Patients With Pulmonary Tuberculosis Resistant to Isoniazid and Rifampin," *New England Journal of Medicine* 328(8):527-532, 1993.
119. Goldberger, M., Supervisory Medical Officer, Division of Antiviral Drug Products, Food and Drug Administration, Public Health Service, U.S. Department of Health and Human Services, Rockville, MD, personal communication, April 1993.
120. Goldberger, M., Supervisory Medical Officer, Division of Antiviral Drug Products, Food and Drug Administration, Public Health Service, U.S. Department of Health and Human Services, Rockville, MD, personal communication, June 4, 1993.
121. Goldberger, M.J., "Tuberculosis Symposium: Emerging Problems and Promise," *Journal of Infectious Diseases* 168(3):537-551, September 1993.
122. Good, R.C., "Serologic Methods for Diagnosing Tuberculosis," *Annals of Internal Medicine* 110(2):97-98, 1989.
123. Good, R.C., and Mastro, T.D., "The Modern Mycobacteriology Laboratory. How It Can Help the Clinician," *Clinics in Chest Medicine* 10(3):315-322, 1989.
124. Gostin, L.O., "Controlling the Resurgent Tuberculosis Epidemic. A 50-State Survey of TB Statutes and Proposals for Reform," *Journal of the American Medical Association* 269(2):255-261, 1993.
125. Gostin, L.O., Executive Director, American Society of Law, Medicine, and Ethics, Boston, MA, personal communication, Mar. 23, 1993.
126. Graham, N.M.H., Nelson, K.E., Solomon, L., et al., "Prevalence of Tuberculin Positivity and Skin Test Anergy in HIV-1-Seropositive and-Seronegative Intravenous Drug Users," *Journal of the American Medical Association* 267(3): 369-373, 1992.
127. Grosset, J., "Present and New Drug Regimens in Chemotherapy and Chemoprophylaxis of Tuberculosis," *Bulletin of the International Union Against Tuberculosis Lung Disease* 65(2-3):86-91, 1990.
128. Hamburg, M.A., "The Challenge of Controlling Tuberculosis in New York City," *New York State Journal of Medicine* 92(7):291-293, 1992.
129. Hamburg, M.A., Commissioner of Health, New York City Department of Health, New York, NY, personal communication to the "Policy Issues in the Control of Tuberculosis" workshop sponsored by the Office of Technology Assessment, U.S. Congress, Washington, DC, Mar. 23, 1993.
130. Hamburg, M.A., Commissioner of Health, New York City Department of Health, New York, NY, statement in hearing before the Subcommittee on Health and the Environment, Committee on Energy and Commerce, House of Representatives, U.S. Congress, Washington, DC, Mar. 29, 1993.
131. Hanson, C.A., and Reichman, L.B., "Tuberculosis Skin Testing and Preventive Therapy," *Seminars in Respiratory Infections* 4(3):182-188, 1989.
132. Harries, A.D., "Tuberculosis and Human Immunodeficiency Virus Infection in Developing Countries," *Lancet* 335:387-390, 1990.
133. Heifets, L.B., "Rapid Automated Methods (BACTEC system) in Clinical Mycobacteriol-

ogy,'' *Seminars in Respiratory Infections* 1:242-249, 1986.

134. Hershfield, E.S., ''BCG Vaccination: Theoretical and Practical Applications,'' *Bulletin of the International Union Against Tuberculosis Lung Disease* 66(suppl):29-30, 1990/91.
135. Heymann, J., ''Battling the Rising Ride of Tuberculosis: An Approach to the American and African Epidemics,'' Working Paper No. H-92-5, Malcolm Wiener Center for Social Policy, John F. Kennedy School of Government, Harvard University, Cambridge, MA, August 1992.
136. Hinman, A., Acting Director, Division of Tuberculosis Elimination, National Center for Prevention Services, Centers for Disease Control, Public Health Service, U.S. Department of Health and Human Services, data summarized in a memo to the Office of Technology Assessment, U.S. Congress, Washington, DC, Sept. 4, 1992.
137. Holloway, C., Director, Office of Science Policy, National Center for Research Resources, National Institutes of Health, Public Health Service, U.S. Department of Health and Human Services, Rockville, MD, personal communication, April 1993.
138. Hong Kong Chest Service, ''A Double-Bind Placebo-Controlled Clinical Trial of Three Antituberculous Chemoprophylaxis Regimens in Patients With Silicosis in Hong Kong, *American Review of Respiratory Disease* 145:36-41, 1992.
139. Hotchkiss, R.L., Directly Observed Treatment of Tuberculosis'' (letter) *New England Journal of Medicine* 329(2):135, 1993.
140. Hotchkiss, R.L., Medical Director, Tuberculosis Program, Mississippi Department of Health, Jackson, MS, personal communication, June 1993.
141. Houde, C., and Dery, P., ''*Mycobacterium bovis sepsis* in an Infant With Human Immunodeficiency Virus Infection,'' *Pediatric Infectious Disease Journal* 7:810-811, 1988.
142. Hsu, K.H.K., ''Thirty Years After Isoniazid. Its Impact on Tuberculosis in Children and Adolescents,'' *Journal of the American Medical Association* 251:1283-1285, 1984.
143. Huebner, R.E., Villarino, M.E., and Snider, D.E., Jr., ''Tuberculin Skin Testing and the HIV Epidemic,'' *Journal of the American Medical Association* 267(3):409-410, 1992.
144. Hutton, M.D., Stead, W.W., Cauthen, G.M., et al., ''Nosocomial Transmission of Tuberculosis Associated With a Draining Abscess,'' *Journal of Infectious Diseases* 161:286-295, 1990.
145. Ingol, D., Director, Office of Affordable Housing and Technology Research, U.S. Department of Housing and Urban Development, Washington, DC, personal communication, June 30, 1993.
146. Institute of Medicine, *The Future of Public Health* (Washington, DC: National Academy Press, 1988).
147. Institute of Medicine, Division of Health Science Policy and Division of International Health, Committee on Emerging Microbial Threats to Health, *Emerging Infections: Microbial Threats to Health in the United States* (Washington, DC: National Academy Press, 1992).
148. International Union Against Tuberculosis Committee on Prophylaxis, ''Efficacy of Various Durations of Isoniazid Preventive Therapy for Tuberculosis: Five Years of Follow-up in the IUAT Trial,'' *Bulletin of the World Health Organization* 60:555-564, 1982.
149. Iseman, M.D., ''Short-Course Chemotherapy of Tuberculosis: The Harsh Realities,'' *Seminars in Respiratory Infections* 1(4):213-219, 1986.
150. Iseman, M.D., ''Less Is More: Short-Course Preventive Therapy of Tuberculosis,'' *American Review of Respiratory Disease* 140:1187, 1989.
151. Iseman, M.D., ''A Leap of Faith. What Can We Do To Curtail Intrainstitutional Transmission of Tuberculosis?'' *Annals of Internal Medicine* 117:251-253, 1992.
152. Iseman, M.D., Professor and Chief, Clinical Mycobacteria Service, School of Medicine, University of Colorado, Denver, CO, personal communication, June 3, 1993.
153. Iseman, M.D., and Madsen, L.A., ''Drug-Resistant Tuberculosis,'' *Clinics in Chest Med-*

icine 10(3):341-353, 1989.

154. Iseman, M.D., and Sbarbaro, J.A., "Short-Course Chemotherapy of Tuberculosis. Hail Britannia (and Friends)!" *American Review of Respiratory Disease* 143:697-698, 1991.
155. Iseman, M.D., and Sbarbaro, J.A., "Compliance and Tuberculosis Treatment," (letter) *Lancet* 337:1609, 1991.
156. Iseman, M.D., and Sbarbaro, J.A., "The Increasing Prevalence of Resistance to Antituberculous Chemotherapeutic Agents: Implications for Global Tuberculosis Control," *Current Clinical Topics in Infectious Diseases* 12:188-207, 1992.
157. Iseman, M.D., Cohn, D.L., and Sbarbaro, J.A., "Directly Observed Treatment of Tuberculosis. We Can't Afford Not to Try It," (editorial) *New England Journal of Medicine* 328(8):576-578, 1993.
158. Jacobs, W.R., Barletta, R.G., Udani, R., et al., "Rapid Assessment of Drug Susceptibilities of Mycobacterium Tuberculosis by Means of Luciferase Reporter Pages," *Science* 260:819-822, 1993.
159. Jereb, J.A., Kelly, G.D., Dooley, S.W., et al., "Tuberculosis Morbidity in the United States: Final Data, 1990," *Morbidity and Mortality Weekly Report* 40(SS-3):23-27, 1991.
160. Jindini, A., Aber, V.R., Edwards, E.A., et al., "The Early Bactericidal Activity of Drugs in Patients With Pulmonary Tuberculosis," *American Review of Respiratory Disease* 121:939, 1980.
161. Johannes, P., Communicable Disease Coordinator, Indian Health Service, Health Resources Services Administration, Public Health Service, U.S. Department of Health and Human Services, Albuquerque, NM, personal communication, April 1993 and June 7, 1993.
162. Johnson, M.P., and Chaisson, R.E., "Tuberculosis and HIV Disease," *AIDS Clinical Review* :109-126, 1991.
163. Jones, D.S., Malecki, J.M., Bigler, W.J., et al., "Pediatric Tuberculosis and Human Immunodeficiency Virus Infection in Palm Beach County, Florida," *American Journal on Diseases of Children* 146:1166-1170, 1992.
164. Jordan, T.J., Lewit, E.M., and Reichman, L.B., "Isoniazid Preventive Therapy for Tuberculosis. Decision Analysis Considering Ethnicity and Gender," *American Review of Respiratory Disease* 144:1357-1360, 1991.
165. Jordan, T.J., Lewit, E.M., Montgomery, R.L., et al., "Isoniazid as Preventive Therapy in HIV-Infected Intravenous Drug Abusers," *Journal of the American Medical Association* 265(22): 2987-2991, 1991.
166. Jordan, W.S., "The Need for a Better Tuberculosis Vaccine," National Vaccine Program Office, U.S. Department of Health and Human Services, Washington, DC, 1992.
167. Kirschstein, R., Director, National Institute of General Medical Science, National Institutes of Health, Bethesda, MD, personal communication, April 1993.
168. Klein, S.J., Acting Director, Division of Epidemiology, New York State Department of Health, Albany, NY, personal communication, June 30, 1993.
169. Koch, R., "Die Aetiologie der Tuberculose," *Berliner klinische Wochenschrift* XIX:221, 1882.
170. Koch-Weser, D., Barrett-Connor, E.L., Comstock, G.W., et al., "BCG Vaccine (Statement of the National Consensus Conference on Tuberculosis)," *Chest* 87(2)(suppl.):133S-134S, 1985.
171. Kochi, A., "The Global Tuberculosis Situation and the New Control Strategy of the World Health Organization," (editorial) *Tubercle* 72(1):1-6, March 1991.
172. Kopanoff, D.E., Kilburn, J.O., Glassroth, J.L., et al., "A Continuing Survey of Tuberculosis Primary Drug Resistance in the United States: March 1975 to November 1977," *American Review of Respiratory Disease* 118:835-842, 1978.
173. Kopanoff, D.E., Snider, D.E. Jr., and Johnson, M., "Recurrent Tuberculosis: Why Do Patients Develop Disease Again? A United States Public Health Service Cooperative Survey," *American Journal of Public Health* 78(1):30-33, 1988.
174. Kramer, F., Modilevsky, T., Waliany, A.R., et al., "Delayed Diagnosis of Tuberculosis in Patients With Human Immunodeficiency Virus

Infection,'' *American Journal of Medicine* 89:451-456, 1990.

175. Lawrence, L., Survey Statistician, Division of Health Care Statistics, National Center for Health Statistics, U.S. Department of Health and Human Services, Hyattsville, MD, personal communication, Apr. 6, 1993.
176. Lederberg, J., Shope, R.E., Oaks, S.C. (eds.), Committee on Emerging Microbial Threats to Health, Division of Health Science Policy and Division of International Health, Institute of Medicine, *Emerging Infections: Microbial Threats to Health in the United States* (Washington, DC: National Academy Press, 1992).
177. Lin, R.Y., and Goodhart, P.T., ''Population Characteristics of Tuberculosis in an HIV/AIDS Registry From an East Harlem Hospital,'' *New York State Journal of Medicine* 91:239-242, 1991.
178. Lordi, G.M., and Reichman, L.B., ''Treatment of Tuberculosis,'' *American Family Physician* 44(1):219-224, 1991.
179. Lotte, A., Was-Hockert, O., Poisson, N., et al., ''Second IUATLD Study on Complications Introduced by Intradermal BCG-Vaccination,'' *Bulletin of the International Union Against Tuberculosis Lung Disease* 63(2):47-59, 1988.
180. Loudon, R.G., and Spohn, S.K., ''Cough Frequency and Infectivity in Patients With Pulmonary Tuberculosis,'' *American Review of Respiratory Disease* 99:109, 1969.
181. Luoto, J., Medical Officer, Office of Refugee Health, Public Health Service, U.S. Department of Health and Human Services, Rockville, MD, personal communication, July 1, 1993.
182. Malasky, C., Jordan, T., Potulski, F., et al., ''Occupational Tuberculous Infections Among Pulmonary Physicians in Training,'' *American Review of Respiratory Disease* 142:505-507, 1990.
183. Martinez, R.M., Assistant Director, Health Financing and Policy, General Accounting Office, U.S. Congress, Washington, DC, personal communication, Nov. 19, 1992.
184. McAdam, J.M., Brickner, P.W., Scharer, L.L., et al., ''The Spectrum of Tuberculosis in a New York City Men's Shelter Clinic (1982-1988),'' *Chest* 97:798-805, 1990.
185. McDonald, K.R., Coordinator, Infectious Disease Program, Health Services Division, Federal Bureau of Prisons, Washington, DC, personal communication, Mar. 15, 1990.
186. McDonald, K.R., Coordinator, Infectious Disease Program, Health Services Division, Federal Bureau of Prisons, Washington, DC, personal communication, July 2, 1993.
187. McDonald, R.J., Memon, A.M., and Reichman, L.B., ''Successful Supervised Ambulatory Management of Tuberculosis Treatment Failures,'' *Annals of Internal Medicine* 96:297-302, 1982.
188. McDonough, J.A., Sada, D.E., Sippola, A.A., et al., ''Microplate and Dot Immunoassays for the Serodiagnosis of Tuberculosis,'' *Journal of Laboratory and Clinical Medicine* 120:318-322, 1992.
189. Miller, B., ''Assessment of Anti-Tuberculosis Drug Shortages, U.S., 1991,'' abstract presented at ''World Congress on Tuberculosis,'' Bethesda, MD, November 1992.
190. Miller, B., Medical Adviser, Division of Tuberculosis Elimination, National Center for Prevention Services, Centers for Disease Control and Prevention, Public Health Service, U.S. Department of Health and Human Services, Atlanta, GA, personal communication, Mar. 31, 1993.
191. Miller, B., Medical Adviser, Division of Tuberculosis Elimination, National Center for Prevention Services, Centers for Disease Control and Prevention, Public Health Service, U.S. Department of Health and Human Services, Atlanta, GA, personal communication, June 14, 1993.
192. Mitchison, D.A., ''The Garrod Lecture: Understanding the Chemotherapy of Tuberculosis—Current Problems,'' *Journal of Antimicrobial Chemotherapy* 29:477-493, 1992.
193. Mitchison, D.A., Professor, Department of Bacteriology, Royal Postgraduate Medical School, London, England, personal communication, June 17, 1993.
194. Mitchison, D.A., and Nunn, A.J., ''Influence of Initial Drug Resistance on the Response to Short-Course Chemotherapy of Pulmonary Tuberculosis,'' *American Review of Respiratory Disease* 133:423-430, 1986.

195. Monno, L., Carbonara, S., Costa, D. et al., "Emergence of Drug-Resistant Mycobacterium Tuberculosis in HIV-Infected Patients," (letter) *Lancet* 337:852, 1991.

196. Moree, M., American Association for the Advancement of Science Fellow, Office of Health, U.S. Agency for International Development, Arlington, VA, personal communication, July 2, 1993.

197. Moree, M., American Association for the Advancement of Science Fellow, Office of Health, U.S. Agency for International Development, Arlington, VA, personal communication, July 7, 1993.

198. Mosteller, F., Professor, School of Public Health, Harvard University, Boston, MA, personal communication, May 1993.

199. Murray, C.J.L., Stylbo, K., and Rouillon, A., "Tuberculosis in Developing Countries: Burden, Intervention and Cost," *Bulletin of the International Union Against Tuberculosis Lung Disease* 65:6-24, 1990.

200. Murray, J.F., "The White Plague: Down and Out, or Up and Coming?" *American Review of Respiratory Disease* 140:1788-1795, 1989.

201. Murray, J.F., "Tuberculosis and Human Immunodeficiency Virus Infection During the 1990's," *Bulletin of the International Union Against Tuberculosis Lung Disease* 66:21-25, 1991.

202. Narain, J.P., Raviglione, M.C., and Kochi, A., "HIV-Associated Tuberculosis in Developing Countries: Epidemiology and Strategies for Prevention," WHO/TB/92.166 (Geneva, Switzerland: World Health Organization, 1992).

203. Narain, J.P., Slutkin, G., ten Dam, H.G., et al., "Preventive Tuberculosis Chemotherapy in HIV Infection: A Priority for Study," *AIDS* 6(7):744-746, 1992.

204. Nardell, E.A., "Dodging Droplet Nuclei. Reducing the Probability of Nosocomial Tuberculosis Transmission in the AIDS Era," *American Review of Respiratory Disease* 142:501-503, 1990.

205. Nardell, E.A., Tuberculosis Control Officer, Division of Tuberculosis Control, State Laboratory Institute, Massachusetts Department of Health, Boston, MA, personal communication, April 1993.

206. Nardell, E.A., Iseman, M.D., Kubica, G., et al., "Multidrug-Resistant Tuberculosis," (letter) *New England Journal of Medicine* 327(16):1173, 1992.

207. Nardell, E., McInnis, B., Thomas, B., et al., "Exogenous Reinfection with Tuberculosis in a Shelter for the Homeless," *New England Journal of Medicine* 315(25):1570-1575, 1986.

208. Nazar-Stewart, V., and Nolan, C.M., "Results of a Directly Observed Intermittent Isoniazid Preventive Therapy Program in a Shelter for Homeless Men," *American Review of Respiratory Disease* 146:57-60, 1992.

209. New York City Task Force on Tuberculosis in the Criminal Justice System, *Final Report*, New York, NY, June 1992.

210. Ninane, J., Grymonprez, A., Burtonboy, G., et al., "Disseminated BCG in HIV Infection," *Archives of Disease in Childhood* 63:1268-1269, 1988.

211. Noble, R.C., "Infectiousness of Pulmonary Tuberculosis After Starting Chemotherapy. Review of the Available Data on an Unresolved Question," *American Journal of Infectious Control* 9:6-10, 1981.

212. Nolan, C.M., "Failure of Therapy for Tuberculosis in Human Immunodeficiency Virus Infection," *American Journal of the Medical Sciences* 304(3):168-173, 1992.

213. Nolan, C.M., Elarth, A.M., Barr, H., et al., "An Outbreak of Tuberculosis in a Shelter for Homeless Men: A Description of Its Evolution and Control," *American Review of Respiratory Disease* 143:257-261, 1991.

214. Novick, A., "Tuberculosis and HIV-Infected Providers," *AIDS Public Policy Journal* 7(2):67-70, 1992.

215. Nunn, P., Githui, W., and Gathua, S., "Tuberculosis and HIV Infection in Kenya," (letter) *Annals Internal of Medicine* 114(3):252-253, 1991

216. O'Brien, R.J., "Present Chemotherapy of Tuberculosis," *Seminars in Respiratory Infections* 4(3):216-224, 1989.

217. O'Brien, R.J., "The Treatment of Tuberculosis," *Tuberculosis: A Comprehensive International Approach*, L.B. Reichman and E.S.

Hershfield (eds.)(New York, NY: Marcel Dekker, Inc., 1993).

218. Onorato, I.M., and McCray, E., "Prevalence of Human Immunodeficiency Virus Infection Among Patients Attending Tuberculosis Clinics in the United States," *Journal of Infectious Diseases* 165:87-92, 1992.

219. Otten, J., Chan, J., and Cleary, T., "Successful Control of an Outbreak of Multidrug-Resistant Tuberculosis in an Urban Teaching Hospital" abstract presented at "World Congress on Tuberculosis," Bethesda, MD, Nov. 16-19, 1992.

220. Passannante, M.R., Restifo, R.A., and Reichman, L.B., "Preventive Therapy for the Patient With Both Universal Indication and Contraindication for Isoniazid," *Chest* 103:825-831, 1993.

221. Patton, L.T., Director, Division of User Liaison, Center for Research Dissemination and Liaison, Agency for Health Care Policy and Research, Public Health Service, U.S. Department of Health and Human Services, Rockville, MD, personal communication, April 1993.

222. Patton, L.T., Director, Division of User Liaison, Center for Research Dissemination and Liaison, Agency for Health Care Policy and Research, Public Health Service, U.S. Department of Health and Human Services, Rockville, MD, personal communication, Aug. 24, 1993.

223. Pearson, M.L., "Nosocomial Transmission of Multidrug-Resistant Mycobacterium Tuberculosis. A Risk to Patients and Health Care Workers," *Journal of the American Medical Association* 117(3):191-196, 1992.

224. Peloquin, C.A., "Shortages of Antimycobacterial Drugs," (letter) *New England Journal of Medicine* 326(10):714, 1992.

225. Pendergast, M.K., Deputy Commissioner and Senior Advisory to the Commissioner, Office of the Commissioner, Food and Drug Administration, Public Health Service, U.S. Department of Health and Human Services, "U.S. Government Incentives for New Technology Development," abstract presented at "World Congress on Tuberculosis," Bethesda, MD, Nov. 18, 1992.

226. Pendergast, M.K., Deputy Commissioner and Senior Advisor to the Commissioner, Office of the Commissioner, Food and Drug Administration, Public Health Service, U.S. Department of Health and Human Services, personal communication, June 8, 1993.

227. Perez-Stable, E.J., and Hopewell, P.C., "Current Tuberculosis Treatment Regimens. Choosing the Right One for Your Patient," *Clinics in Chest Medicine* 10(3):323-339, 1989.

228. Phelps, J., Program Analyst, Office of Program Planning and Evaluation, National Institute of Environmental Health Sciences, Centers for Disease Control and Prevention, Public Health Service, U.S. Department of Health and Human Services, Research Triangle Park, NC, personal communication, Apr. 14, 1993.

229. Pitchenik, A., Tuberculosis Control and the AIDS Epidemic in Developing Countries," *Annals of Internal Medicine* 113(2):89-91, 1990.

230. Pitchenik, A.E., and Fertel, D., "Tuberculosis and Nontuberculous Mycobacterial Disease," *Medical Clinics of North America* 76(1):121-171, 1992.

231. Pitchenik, A.E., Cole, C., Russell, B.W., et al., "Tuberculosis, Atypical Mycobacteriosis, and the Acquired Immunodeficiency Syndrome Among Haitian and Non-Haitian Patients in South Florida," *Annals of Internal Medicine* 101:641-645, 1984.

232. Pitchenik, A.E., Fertel, D., and Bloch, A.B., "Mycobacterial Disease: Epidemiology, Diagnosis, Treatment and Prevention," *Clinics in Chest Medicine* 9:425-441, 1988.

233. Powell, K.E., and Farer, L.S., "The Rising Age of the Tuberculosis Patient: A Sign of Success and Failure," *Journal of Infectious Diseases* 142(6):946-948, 1980.

234. Price, L.E., Rutala, W.A., and Samsa, G.P., "Tuberculosis in Hospital Personnel," *Infection Control* 8(3):97-101, 1987.

235. Pust, R.E., "Tuberculosis in the 1990s: Resurgence, Regimens, and Resources," *Southern Medical Journal* 85(6):584-593, 1992.

236. Raviglione, M.C., Narain, J.P., Kochi, A., "HIV-Associated Tuberculosis in Developing Countries: Clinical Features, Diagnosis, and

Treatment,'' *Bulletin of the International Union Against Tuberculosis Lung Disease* 70(4):515-526, 1992.

237. Reeves, R., Blakey, D., Snider, D.E., Jr., etal., ''Transmission of Multiple Drug Resistant TB: Report of a School and Community Outbreak,'' *American Journal of Epidemiology* 113:423-435, 1981.

238. Reichman, L.B., ''Why Hasn't BCG Proved Dangerous in HIV-Infected Patients?'' (letter) *Journal of American Medical Association* 261(22):3246, 1989.

239. Reichman, L.B., ''The National Tuberculosis Training Initiative,'' *Annals of Internal Medicine* 111(3):197-198, 1989.

240. Reichman, L.B., ''The U-Shaped Curve of Concern,'' *American Review of Respiratory Disease* 144(4):741-742, 1991.

241. Reichman, L.B., ''Dealing With the Resurgence of Tuberculosis,'' (editorial) *American Family Physician* 43(2):448, 1991.

242. Reichman, L.B., ''HIV Infection: The Dominant New Face of Tuberculosis,'' *Mount Sinai Journal of Medicine* 59(3):271-277, 1992.

243. Reichman, L.B., President, American Lung Association, New York, NY, personal communication to the ''Policy Issues in the Control of Tuberculosis'' workshop sponsored by the Office of Technology Assessment, Washington, DC, Mar. 23, 1993.

244. Reichman, L.B., President, American Lung Association, New York, NY, statement in hearing before the Subcommittee on Health and the Environment, Committee on Energy and Commerce, House of Representatives, U.S. Congress, Washington, DC, Mar. 29, 1993.

245. Reichman, L.B., and O'Day, R., ''Tuberculous Infection in a Large Urban Population,'' *American Review of Respiratory Disease* 117:705-712, 1978.

246. Reichman, L.B., Felton, C.P., and Edsall, J.R., ''Drug Dependence, A Possible New Risk Factor for Tuberculosis Disease,'' *Archives of Internal Medicine* 139:337-339, 1979.

247. Richmond, L., Assistant to the Director, Montefiore-Rikers Island Health Services, Montefiore Medical Center, The University Hospital for the Albert Einstein College of Medicine, New York, NY, personal communication, June 21, 1993.

248. Rieder, H.L., and Snider, D.E., Jr., ''Tuberculosis and the Acquired Immunodeficiency Syndrome,'' (editorial) *Chest* 90:469-470, 1986.

249. Rieder, H.L., Cauthen, G.M., Comstock, G.W., et al., ''Epidemiology of Tuberculosis in the United States,'' *Epidemiologic Reviews* 11:79-98, 1989.

250. Rieder, H.L., Kelly, G.D., Bloch, A.B., et al., ''Tuberculosis Diagnosed at Death in the United States,'' *Chest* 100:678-811, 1991.

251. Rieder, H.L., Snider, D.E., Jr., and Cauthen, G.M., ''Extrapulmonary Tuberculosis in the United States,'' *American Review of Respiratory Disease* 141:347-351, 1990.

252. Riley, R.L., and Nardell, E.A., ''Clearing the Air. The Theory and Application of Ultraviolet Air Disinfection,'' *American Review of Respiratory Disease* 139:1286-1294, 1989.

253. Riley, R.L., Mills, C.C., O'Grady, F., et al., ''Infectiousness of Air From a Tuberculosis Ward. Ultraviolet Irradiation of Infected Air: Comparative Infectiousness of Different Patients,'' *American Review of Respiratory Disease* 85:511-525, 1962.

254. Roper, W.L., ''Issues in Preventing Tuberculosis Transmission in Health Care Facilities,'' transcript of presentation delivered at the Centers for Disease Control, Public Health Service, U.S. Department of Health and Human Services, Atlanta, GA, Oct. 23, 1992.

255. Roper, W.L., Director, Centers for Disease Control and Prevention, Public Health Service, U.S. Department of Health and Human Services, statement in hearing before the Subcommittee on Health and the Environment, Committee on Energy and Commerce, House of Representatives, U.S. Congress, Washington, DC, Mar. 29, 1993.

256. Rose, D.N., Schecter, C.B., and Silver, A.L., ''The Age Threshold for Isoniazid Chemoprophylaxis: A Decision Analysis for Low-Risk Tuberculin Reactors,'' *Journal of the American Medical Association* 256:2709-2713, 1986.

257. Roselle, G.A., Medical Service, Central Office, U.S. Department of Veterans Affairs, Cincin-

nati, OH, "Infection Control," mimeograph, May 28, 1992.

258. Roselle, G.A., Program Director for Infectious Diseases, U.S. Department of Veterans Affairs, Cincinnati, OH, "Tuberculosis Cases—National Infection Control Survey Results," memorandum to the Director, Medical Service, Central Office, U.S. Department of Veterans Affairs, Cincinnati, OH, Jan. 6, 1993.
259. Roselle, G.A., Denny, F., Danko, L.H., Reviewers, East Orange Veterans Affairs Medical Center tuberculosis outbreak site, "East Orange VMAC report," memorandum to the Director, Medical Service, Central Office, U.S. Department of Veterans Affairs and to the Director, Office of Occupational Safety and Health, U.S. Department of Veterans Affairs, Cincinnati, OH, Oct. 14, 1992.
260. Rosenberg, Z., Assistant to the Director, National Institute of Allergy and Infectious Diseases, National Institutes of Health, Public Health Service, U.S. Department of Health and Human Services, Bethesda, MD, personal communication, June 4, 1993.
261. Rosenberg, Z., Assistant to the Director, National Institute for Allergy and Infectious Diseases, National Institutes of Health, Public Health Service, U.S. Department of Health and Human Services, Bethesda, MD, personal communication, July 14, 1993; based on data from P. Wexler, Budget Analyst, Budget Office, National Institutes of Health, Public Health Service, U.S. Department of Health and Human Services, Bethesda, MD.
262. Rouillon, A., and Ogasawara, F.R., "The Role of Nongovernmental Organizations," *Tuberculosis: A Comprehensive International Approach*, L.B. Reichman and E.S. Hershfield (eds.)(New York, NY: Marcel Dekker, Inc., 1993).
263. Rubel, A.J., and Garro, L.C., "Social and Cultural Factors in the Successful Control of Tuberculosis," *Public Health Reports* 107(6):626-636, 1992.
264. Salomon, P., Acting Chief Medical Officer, Primary Health Care, Administrator's Office, Health Resources and Services Administration, Public Health Service, U.S. Department of Health and Human Services, personal communication, June 30, 1993.
265. Sbarbaro, J.A., "Compliance: Inducements and Enforcements," *Chest* 76(6):750-756, 1979.
266. Sbarbaro, J.A., "Public Health Aspects of Tuberculosis: Supervision of Therapy," *Clinics in Chest Medicine* 1(2):253-263, 1980.
267. Sbarbaro, J.A., "Reality Versus the Academic Milieu," *American Review of Respiratory Disease* 134:1109, 1986.
268. Sbarbaro, J.A., "Skin Testing in the Diagnosis of Tuberculosis," *Seminars in Respiratory Infections* 1(4):234-238, 1986.
269. Sbarbaro, J.A., "The Patient-Physician Relationship: Compliance Revisited," *Annals of Allergy* 64:325-331, 1990.
270. Sbarbaro, J.A., "The Plan To Eliminate Tuberculosis in the United States," *Tuberculosis: A Comprehensive International Approach*, L.B. Reichman and E.S. Hershfield (eds.)(New York, NY: Marcel Dekker, Inc., 1993).
271. Sbarbaro, J.A., and Iseman, M.D., "Baby Needs a New Pair of Shoes," *Chest* 90(5):754-755, 1986.
272. Sbarbaro, J.A., and Johnson, S., "Tuberculosis Chemotherapy for Recalcitrant Outpatients Administered Twice Weekly," *American Review of Respiratory Disease* 96:895-902, 1968.
273. Sbarbaro, J.A., Barlow, P., and Craig, M., "Intermittent Chemotherapy for Adults With Tuberculosis," *American Review of Respiratory Disease* 110:374, 1974.
274. Schecter, G., Tuberculosis Controller, Department of Public Health, City and County of San Francisco, CA, personal communication to the "Policy Issues in the Control of Tuberculosis" workshop sponsored by the Office of Technology Assessment, Washington, DC, Mar. 23, 1993.
275. Schieffelbein, C.W., and Snider, D.E., Jr., "Tuberculosis Control Among Homeless Populations," *Archives of Internal Medicine* 148:1843-1846, 1988.
276. Schweinle, J.E., "Evolving Concepts of the Epidemiology, Diagnosis, and Therapy of Mycobacterium Tuberculosis Infection," *Yale Journal of Biology and Medicine* 63:565-579, 1990.

277. Selwyn, P.A., "Tuberculosis in the AIDS Era: A New Threat From an Old Disease," *New York State Journal of Medicine* 91:233-235, 1991.

278. Selwyn, P.A., Hartel, D., Lewis, V.A., et al., "A Prospective Study of the Risk of Tuberculosis Among Intravenous Drug Users With Human Immunodeficiency Virus Infection," *New England Journal of Medicine* 320:545-550, 1989.

279. Selwyn, P.A., Sckell, B.M., Alcabes, P., et al., "High Risk of Active Tuberculosis in HIV-Infected Drug Users With Cutaneous Anergy," *Journal of the American Medical Association* 268(4):504-509, 1992.

280. Shafer, R.W., Kelly, P., Larkin, C., et al., "Multidrug-Resistant TB at a New York City Hospital," abstract presented at "World Congress on Tuberculosis," Bethesda MD, November 1992.

281. Shankar, P., Manjunath, N., Lakshmi, R., et al., "Identification of Mycobacterium Tuberculosis by Polymerase Chain Reaction," *Lancet* 335:423, 1990.

282. Shaw, S., Medicaid State Representative, Division of Medicaid, Health Care Financing Administration, U.S. Department of Health and Human Services, New York, NY, personal communication, Mar. 30, 1993.

283. Shaw, S., Medicaid State Representative, Division of Medicaid, Health Care Financing Administration, U.S. Department of Health and Human Services, New York, NY, personal communication, Apr. 5, 1993.

284. Shaw, S., Medicaid State Representative, Division of Medicaid, Health Care Financing Administration, U.S. Department of Health and Human Services, New York, NY, personal communication, June 14, 1993.

285. Sherman, M.N., Brickner, P.W., Schwartz, M.S., et al., "Tuberculosis in Single-Room-Occupancy Hotel Residents: A Persisting Focus of Disease," *New York Medical Quarterly* 2:39-41, 1980.

286. Siegfried, J.D., Associate Vice President for Medical Affairs, Pharmaceutical Manufacturers Association, Washington, DC, personal communication, June 7, 1993.

287. Simone, P.M., and Iseman, M.D., "Drug-Resistant Tuberculosis: A Deadly—and Growing—Danger," *Journal of Respiratory Diseases* 13(7):960-971, 1992.

288. Sloand, E., Special Assistant to the Director, National Heart, Lung, and Blood Institute, National Institutes of Health, Public Health Service, U.S. Department of Health and Human Services, personal communication, Apr. 1, 1993.

289. Slutkin, G., "Management of Tuberculosis Among Urban Homeless Indigents," *Public Health Reports* 101(5):481-485, 1986.

290. Small, P.M., Schecter, G.F., Goodman P.C., et al., "Treatment of Tuberculosis in Patients With Advanced Human Immunodeficiency Virus Infection," *New England Journal of Medicine* 324:289-294, 1991.

291. Snider, D.E., Jr., "Bacilli Calmette-Guerin Vaccinations and Tuberculin Skin Tests," *Journal of the American Medical Association* 253(23):3438-3439, 1985.

292. Snider, D.E., Jr., "Decision Analysis for Isoniazid Preventive Therapy: Take It or Leave It?" *American Review of Respiratory Disease* 137:2-3, 1988.

293. Snider, D.E., Jr., "The Impact of Tuberculosis on Women, Children, and Minorities in the United States," paper presented at "World Congress on Tuberculosis," Bethesda, MD, November 1992.

294. Snider, D.E., Jr., and Caras, G.J., "Isoniazid-Associated Hepatitis Deaths: A Review of Available Information," *American Review of Respiratory Disease* 145:494-497, 1992.

295. Snider, D.E., Jr., Salinas, L., and Kelly, G.D., "Tuberculosis: An Increasing Problem Among Minorities in the United States," *Public Health Reports* 104:645-654, 1989.

296. Snider, D.E., Jr., Seggerson, J.J., and Hutton, M.D., "Tuberculosis and Migrant Farm Workers," *Journal of the American Medical Association* 265(13):1732, 1991.

297. Snider, D.E., Jr., Cauthen, G.M., Farer, L.S., et al., "Drug-Resistant Tuberculosis" (letter) *American Review of Respiratory Disease* 144:732, 1991.

298. Snider, D.E., Jr., Kelly, G.D., Cauthen, G.M., et al., "Infection and Disease Among Contacts of Tuberculosis Cases With Drug-Resistant and Drug-Susceptible Bacilli," *American Review of Respiratory Disease* 132:125-132, 1985.
299. Sontag, S., *Illness as Metaphor and AIDS and Its Metaphors* (New York, NY: Doubleday, 1990).
300. Starke, J.R., "Prevention of Tuberculosis," *Seminars in Respiratory Infections* 4(4):318-325, 1989.
301. Starke, J.R., "Multidrug Therapy for Tuberculosis in Children," *Pediatric Infectious Disease Journal* 9:785-793, 1990.
302. Starke, J.R., "Current Concepts of Epidemiology, Diagnosis and Treatment of Childhood Tuberculosis in the United States," *Indian Pediatrics* 28(4):335-355, 1991.
303. Starke, J.R., "Current Chemotherapy for Tuberculosis in Children," *Infectious Disease Clinics of North America* 6:215-238, 1992.
304. Starke, J.R., Assistant Professor of Medicine, School of Medicine, Baylor University, Waco, TX, personal communication, Mar. 23, 1993.
305. Starke, J.R., and Connelly, K.K., "Bacilli Calmette-Guerin (BCG) Vaccine," Baylor University, Waco, TX, unpublished manuscript, 1992.
306. Starke, J.R., and Taylor-Watts, K.T., "Tuberculosis in the Pediatric Population of Houston, Texas," *Pediatrics* 84:28-35, 1989.
307. Starke, J.R., Jacobs, R.F., Jereb, J., "Resurgence of Tuberculosis in Children," *Journal of Pediatrics* 120(6):839-855, 1992.
308. Stead, W.W., "Undetected Tuberculosis in Prison. Source of Infection for the Community at Large," *Journal of the American Medical Association* 240:2544-2547, 1978.
309. Stead, W.W., "Special Problems in Tuberculosis," *Clinics in Chest Medicine* 10(3):397-406, 1989.
310. Stead, W.W., "Skin Ulcers and Tuberculosis Outbreaks," (letter) *Annals of Internal Medicine* 118(6):474, 1993.
311. Stead, W.W., and Dutt, A.K., "Tuberculosis in Elderly Persons," *Annual Review of Medicine* 42:267-276, 1991.
312. Stead, W.W., Lofgren, J.P., and Warren, E., "Tuberculosis as an Endemic and Nosocomial Infection Among the Elderly in Nursing Homes," *New England Journal of Medicine* 312:1483-1487, 1985.
313. Stover, C.K., de la Cruz, V.F., Fuerst, T.R., et al., "New Use of BCG for Recombinant Vaccines," *Nature* 351:456-460, 1991.
314. Stover, E., Director, Office on AIDS, National Institute of Mental Health, National Institutes of Health, Public Health Service, U.S. Department of Health and Human Services, Bethesda, MD, personal communication, Apr. 1993.
315. Styblo, K., "The Impact of HIV Infection on the Global Epidemiology of Tuberculosis," *Bulletin of the International Union Against Tuberculosis and Lung Disease* 66:27-32, 1991.
316. Sudre, P., tenDam, G., Kochi, A., "Tuberculosis: A Global Overview of the Situation Today," *Bulletin of the World Health Organization* 70(2):149-159, 1992.
317. Sumartojo, E., "When Tuberculosis Treatment Fails: A Social Behavioral Account of Patient Adherence," *American Review of Respiratory Disease* 147:1311-1320, 1993.
318. Sumartojo, E., Research Psychologist, Division of Tuberculosis Elimination, National Center for Prevention Services, Center Disease Control, Public Health Service, U.S. Department of Health and Human Service, personal communication, June 1993.
319. Sunderam, G., McDonald, R.J., Maniatis, T., et al., "Tuberculosis as a Manifestation of the Acquired Immunodeficiency Syndrome (AIDS)," *Journal of American Medical Association* 256(3):362-366, 1986.
320. Taylor, W.C., Aronson, M.D., and Delbanco, T.L., "Should Young Adults with a Positive Tuberculin Test Take Isoniazid?" *Annals of Internal Medicine* 94:808-813, 1981.
321. Theuer, C.D., Hopewell, P.C., Elias, D., et al., "Human Immunodeficiency Virus Infection in Tuberculosis Patients," *Journal of Infectious Disease* 162:8-12, 1990.
322. Thierry, D., Chureau, C., Aznar, C., et al., "The Detection of Mycobacterium Tuberculosis in Uncultured Clinical Specimens Using the Polym-

erase Chain Reaction and a Non-Radioactive DNA Probe,'' *Molecular and Cellular Probes* 6:181-191, 1992.

323. Thorburn, K.M., Immediate Past President, American Correctional Health Services Association, Honolulu, HI, personal communication, June 8, 1993.
324. Tokars, J.I., Jarvis, W.R., Edlin, B.R., et al., ''Tuberculin Skin Testing of Hospital Employees During an Outbreak of Multidrug-Resistant Tuberculosis in Human Immunodeficiency Virus (HIV)-Infected Patients,'' (letter) *Infection Control and Hospital Epidemiology* 13(9):509-510, 1992.
325. Torres, R.A., Mani, S., Altholz, J., et al., ''Human Immunodeficiency Virus Infection Among Homeless Men in a New York City Shelter: Association With Mycobacterium Tuberculosis Infection,'' *Archives of Internal Medicine* 150:2030-2036, 1990.
326. Tubercle, ''Defaulters and Motivation'' (editorial) *Tubercle* 53:147-148, 1972.
327. Tuberculosis Prevention Trial, Mendis, ''Trial of BCG Vaccines in South India for Tuberculous Infection,'' *Indian Journal of Medical Research* 1972(suppl.):1-74, 1980.
328. Underwood, M.A., Berg, R., Bryant, J.K., et al., Association of Practitioners in Infection Control, Guidelines Committee, ''Commentary From the APIC Guidelines Committee on the Centers for Disease Control 'Guidelines for Preventing the Transmission of Tuberculosis in Health-Care Settings, With Special Focus on HIV-Related Issues,''' *American Journal of Infection Control* 20(1):27-29, 1992.
329. U.S. Congress, Office of Technology Assessment, *Evaluation of the Oregon Medicaid Proposal*, OTA-H-531 (Washington, DC: U.S. Government Printing Office, May 1992).
330. U.S. Department of Health and Human Services, Public Health Service, Centers for Disease Control, ''The Centers for Disease Control History of Tuberculosis Funding FY 1960 to 1993,'' unpublished report, 1993.
331. U.S. Congress, Office of Technology Assessment, *The CDC's Case Definition of AIDS: Implications of the Proposed Revisions. HIV-Related Issues: Background Paper 8*, OTA-BP-H-89 (Washington, DC: U.S. Government Printing Office, August 1992).
332. U.S. Department of Health and Human Services, The Fiscal Year 1994 Budget, unpublished manuscript, Washington, DC, Apr. 8, 1993.
333. U.S. Department of Health and Human Services, National Vaccine Program Office, information sheet, undated.
333a. U.S. Department of Health and Human Services, Public Health Service, Centers for Disease Control, unpublished data, undated.
334. U.S. Department of Health and Human Services, Public Health Service, Centers for Disease Control, ''Tuberculosis Cases and Case Rates: States, 1990 and 1991,'' unpublished table, undated.
334a. U.S. Department of Health and Human Services, Public Health Service, Centers for Disease Control, ''Tuberculosis Cases and Case Rates: Cities of 250,000 or More, 1990 and 1991,'' unpublished table, undated.
334b. U.S. Department of Health and Human Services, Public Health Service, Centers for Disease Control, ''Tuberculosis Cases and Case Rates, Deaths and Death Rates, United States, 1953-1991,'' unpublished table, undated.
335. U.S. Department of Health and Human Services, Public Health Service, Centers for Disease Control, unpublished survey on tuberculosis cases reported from 29 states 1984-85, undated.
336. U.S. Department of Health and Human Services, Public Health Service, Centers for Disease Control and Prevention, ''Tuberculosis Control Laws in the United States: A Survey and Recommendations,'' draft report, Atlanta, GA, Sept. 30, 1992.
337. U.S. Department of Health, Public Health Service, Centers for Disease Control and Prevention, ''Tuberculosis in 1992: A Progress Report,'' Advisory Committee for the Elimination of Tuberculosis, U.S. Department of Health and Human Services, Atlanta, GA, mimeograph, May 15, 1993.
338. U.S. Department of Health and Human Services, Public Health Service, Centers for Disease Control and Prevention, ''Primary Resistance to Antituberculosis Drugs—United States,''

Morbidity and Mortality Weekly Report 29(29): 345-346, 1980.

339. U.S. Department of Health and Human Services, Public Health Service, Centers for Disease Control and Prevention, "Outbreak of Multidrug-Resistant Tuberculosis—Texas, California, and Pennsylvania," *Morbidity and Mortality Weekly Report* 39:369-372, 1990.
340. U.S. Department of Health and Human Services, Public Health Service, Centers for Disease Control and Prevention, "Primary Resistance to Antituberculosis Drugs—United States," *Morbidity and Mortality Weekly Report* 32(40):521-523, 1983.
341. U.S. Department of Health and Human Services, Public Health Service, Centers for Disease Control and Prevention, "Disseminated *Mycobacterium bovis* Infection From BCG Vaccination of a Patient With AIDS," *Morbidity and Mortality Weekly Report* 34:227-228, 1985.
342. U.S. Department of Health and Human Services, Public Health Service, Centers for Disease Control and Prevention, "Tuberculosis Control Among Homeless Populations," *Morbidity and Mortality Weekly Report* 36(17):257-260, 1987.
343. U.S. Department of Health and Human Services, Public Health Service, Centers for Disease Control and Prevention, "Use of BCG Vaccines in the Control of Tuberculosis: A Joint Statement by the ACIP and the Advisory Committee for Elimination of Tuberculosis," *Morbidity and Mortality Weekly Report* 37(43):663-664, 669-675, 1988.
344. U.S. Department of Health and Human Services, Public Health Service, Centers for Disease Control and Prevention, "Tuberculosis and Human Immunodeficiency Virus Infection: Recommendations of the Advisory Committee for Elimination of Tuberculosis (ACET)," *Morbidity and Mortality Weekly Report* 38(14):236-238, 243-250, 1989.
345. U.S. Department of Health and Human Services, Public Health Service, Centers for Disease Control and Prevention, "*Mycobacterium tuberculosis* Transmission in a Health Clinic—Florida, 1988," *Morbidity and Mortality Weekly Report* 38(15):256-258, 263-264, 1989.
346. U.S. Department of Health and Human Services, Public Health Service, Centers for Disease Control and Prevention, "Prevention and Control of Tuberculosis in Correctional Institutions. Recommendations of the Advisory Committee for the Elimination of Tuberculosis," *Morbidity and Mortality Weekly Report* 38(18):313-320, 325, 1989.
347. U.S. Department of Health and Human Services, Public Health Service, Centers for Disease Control and Prevention, "Bovine tuberculosis—Pennsylvania," *Morbidity and Mortality Weekly Report* 39(12):201-203, 1990.
348. U.S. Department of Health and Human Services, Public Health Service, Centers for Disease Control and Prevention, "Transmission of Multidrug-Resistant Tuberculosis From an HIV-Positive Client in a Residential Substance-Abuse Treatment Facility—Michigan," *Morbidity and Mortality Weekly Report* 40(8):129-131, 1991.
349. U.S. Department of Health and Human Services, Public Health Service, Centers for Disease Control, "Crack Cocaine Use Among Persons With Tuberculosis—Contra Costa County, California, 1987-1990," *Morbidity and Mortality Weekly Report* 40(29):485-489, 1991.
350. U.S. Department of Health and Human Services, Public Health Service, Centers for Disease Control and Prevention, "Nosocomial Transmission of Multidrug-Resistant Tuberculosis Among HIV-Infected Persons—Florida and New York, 1988-1991," *Morbidity and Mortality Weekly Report* 40(34):585-591, 1991.
351. U.S. Department of Health and Human Services, Public Health Service, Centers for Disease Control and Prevention, "Tuberculosis Among Residents of Shelters for the Homeless," *Morbidity and Mortality Weekly Report* 40(50):869-871, 877 1991.
352. U.S. Department of Health and Human Services, Public Health Service, Centers for Disease Control and Prevention, "Availability of Streptomycin and Para-Aminosalicylic Acid—United States," *Morbidity and Mortality Weekly Report* 41(14):243, 1992.

352a. U.S. Department of Health and Human Services, Public Health Service, Centers for Disease

Control and Prevention, "Transmission of Multidrug-Resistant Tuberculosis Among Immunocompromised Persons, Correctional System—New York, 1991," *Morbidity and Mortality Weekly Report* 41:507-509, 1992.

353. U.S. Department of Health and Human Services, Public Health Service, Centers for Disease Control and Prevention, "Tuberculosis Morbidity—United States, 1991." *Morbidity and Mortality Weekly Report* 41(14):240, 1992.

354. U.S. Department of Health and Human Services, Public Health Service, Centers for Disease Control and Prevention, "Approaches to Improving Adherence to Antituberculosis Therapy," *Morbidity and Mortality Weekly Report* 42:74-75, 81 1993.

355. U.S. Department of Health and Human Services, Public Health Service, Centers for Disease Control and Prevention, "Tuberculosis Prevention in Drug-Treatment Centers and Correctional Facilities—Selected U.S. Sites, 1990-1991," *Morbidity and Mortality Weekly Report* 42(11):210-213, 1993.

356. U.S. Department of Health and Human Services, Public Health Service, Centers for Disease Control and Prevention, "Tuberculosis Morbidity—United States," *Morbidity and Mortality Weekly Report* 42(18):363, 1993.

357. U.S. Department of Health and Human Services, Public Health Service, Centers for Disease Control and Prevention, "Screening for Tuberculosis and Tuberculous Infection in High-Risk Populations. Recommendations of the Advisory Committee for Elimination of Tuberculosis," *Morbidity and Mortality Weekly Report* 39(RR-8):1-12, 1990.

358. U.S. Department of Health and Human Services, Public Health Service, Centers for Disease Control and Prevention, "Prevention and Control of Tuberculosis in Facilities Providing Long-Term Care to the Elderly. Recommendations of the Advisory Committee for the Elimination of Tuberculosis," *Morbidity and Mortality Weekly Report* 39(RR-10):7-20, 1990.

359. U.S. Department of Health and Human Services, Public Health Service, Centers for Disease Control and Prevention, "Guidelines for Preventing the Transmission of Tuberculosis in Health-Care Settings, With Special Focus on HIV-Related Issues," *Morbidity and Mortality Weekly Report* 39(RR-17):1-29, 1990.

360. U.S. Department of Health and Human Services, Public Health Service, Centers for Disease Control and Prevention, "Tuberculosis Among Foreign-Born Persons Entering the United States. Recommendations of the Advisory Council for the Elimination of Tuberculosis," *Morbidity and Mortality Weekly Report* 39(RR-18):1-21, 1990.

361. U.S. Department of Health and Human Services, Public Health Service, Centers for Disease Control and Prevention, "Purified Protein Derivative (PPD)-Tuberculin Anergy and HIV Infection: Guidelines for Anergy Testing and Management of Anergic Persons at Risk of Tuberculosis," *Morbidity and Mortality Weekly Report* 40(RR-5):27-33, 1991.

362. U.S. Department of Health and Human Services, Public Health Service, Centers for Disease Control and Prevention, "Prevention and Control of Tuberculosis in Migrant Farm Workers. Recommendations of the Advisory Council for the Elimination of Tuberculosis," *Morbidity and Mortality Weekly Report* 41(RR-10):1-14, 1992.

363. U.S. Department of Health and Human Services, Public Health Service, Centers for Disease Control and Prevention, "National Action Plan to Combat Multidrug-Resistant Tuberculosis," *Morbidity and Mortality Weekly Report* 41(RR-11), 1992.

364. U.S. Department of Health and Human Services, Public Health Service, Centers for Disease Control and Prevention, "Revised Classification System for HIV Infection and Expanded Surveillance Case Definition for AIDS Among Adolescents and Adults," *Morbidity and Mortality Weekly Report* 41(RR-17):1-19, 1992.

365. U.S. Department of Health and Human Services, Public Health Service, Centers for Disease Control and Prevention, "Projections of the Number of Persons Diagnosed With AIDS and the Number of Immunosuppressed HIV-Infected Persons," *Morbidity and Mortality Weekly Report* 41(RR-18):1-29, 1992.

366. U.S. Department of Health and Human Services, Public Health Service, Centers for Disease Control and Prevention, "Initial Therapy for Tuberculosis in the Era of Multidrug Resistance. Recommendations of the Advisory Council for the Elimination of Tuberculosis," *Morbidity and Mortality Weekly Report* 42(RR-7):1-8, 1993.
367. U.S. Department of Health and Human Services, Public Health Service, Centers for Disease Control and Prevention, "A Strategic Plan for the Elimination of Tuberculosis in the United States," *Morbidity and Mortality Weekly Report* 38(S-3):1-25, 1989.
368. U.S. Department of Health and Human Services, Public Health Service, Centers for Disease Control, Advisory Council for the Elimination of Tuberculosis, minutes, Atlanta, GA, Sept. 24-25, 1992.
369. U.S. Department of Health and Human Services, Public Health Service, Centers for Disease Control and Prevention, Interagency Tuberculosis Working Groups, "Proposed Steps for Implementing the National Action Plan to Combat Multidrug-Resistant Tuberculosis," U.S. Department of Health and Human Services, unpublished report, Sept. 24, 1992.
370. U.S. Department of Health and Human Services, Public Health Service, Centers for Disease Control and Prevention, National Center for Prevention Services, *Program Briefing, 1992: Tuberculosis Elimination*, U.S. Department of Health and Human Services, Atlanta, GA, unpublished report, Mar. 9, 1993.
371. U.S. Department of Health and Human Services, Public Health Service, Centers for Disease Control and Prevention, National Institute for Occupational Safety and Health, "Recommended Guidelines for Person Respiratory Protection of Workers in Health-Care Facilities Potentially Exposed to Tuberculosis," U.S. Department of Health and Human Services, Washington, DC, Sept. 14, 1992.
372. U.S. Department of Health and Human Services, Public Health Service, National Institutes of Health, National Center for Nursing Research, "Tuberculosis: Prevention and Adherence Interventions," No. RFA: NR-93-004, NIH Guide 22(11), March 19, 1993.
373. U.S. Department of Health and Human Services, Public Health Service, National Institutes of Health, National Institute of Allergy and Infectious Diseases, "Research on Tuberculosis," paper prepared by the Office of Communications, National Institute of Allergy and Infectious Diseases, National Institutes of Health, Public Health Service, U.S. Department of Health and Human Services, Bethesda, MD, November 1992.
374. U.S. Department of Health and Human Services, Public Health Service, National Institutes of Health, National Institute for Allergy and Infectious Diseases, "Research Agenda for Tuberculosis," background monograph prepared by the Office of Communications, National Institute for Allergy and Infectious Diseases, Bethesda, MD, June 1993.
375. U.S. Department of Health and Human Services, Public Health Service, National Institutes of Health, National Institute on Drug Abuse, "The Spread of Tuberculosis Among Drug Users," Program Announcement No. PA-93-44, January 1993.
376. U.S. Department of Health and Human Services, Public Health Service, National Institutes of Health, Office of Science Policy and Legislation, table showing NIH budgets for tuberculosis in fiscal years 1991, 1992, and 1993, Feb. 19, 1993.
377. U.S. Department of Health and Human Services, Social Security Administration, *Disability Evaluation Under Social Security*, SSA Publication No. 64-039 (Washington, DC: U.S. Government Printing Office, May 1992).
378. U.S. Department of Health and Human Services and the American Thoracic Society, *Core Curriculum on Tuberculosis, National Tuberculosis Training Initiative, 2nd Edition* (Atlanta, GA: U.S. Department of Health and Human Services, April 1991).
379. U.S. Department of Veterans Affairs, Veterans Health Administration, "TB Control Responsibilities of VA Facilities," VA Directive No. 10-92-063, Washington, DC, June 4, 1992.

380. Van Scoy, R.E., and Wilkowske, C.J., ''Antituberculous Agents,'' *Mayo Clinic Proceedings* 67:179-187, 1992.

381. Vennema, A., ''Contact Investigation and Isoniazid Chemoprophylaxis in New York City, 1979-1987,'' *New York State Journal of Medicine* 92(2):185-188, 1992.

382. Villarino, M.E., Geiter, L.J., and Simone, P.M., ''The Multidrug-Resistant Tuberculosis Challenge to Public Health Efforts to Control Tuberculosis,'' *Public Health Reports* 107(6):616-625, 1992.

383. Wadhawan, D., Hira, S., Hwansa, N., et al., ''Preventive Tuberculosis Chemotherapy With Isoniazid Among Persons Infected With Human Immunodeficiency Virus,'' (Abstract No. WB 2261:247) presented at ''VII International Conference on AIDS,'' Florence, Italy, 1991.

384. Welch, D.F., Guruswamy, A.P., Shaw, C.W., et al., ''Implications of Multi-Drug Resistant Tuberculosis for Clinical Laboratories,'' as cited in J.L. Cox, ''Coalition Reacts to Surge of Drug-Resistant TB,'' *American Society of Microbiology News* 58:135-139, 1992.

385. Werhane, M.J., Snukst-Torbeck, G., and Schraufnagel, D.E., ''The Tuberculosis Clinic,'' *Chest* 96(4):815-818, 1989.

386. World Health Organization, ''Expanded Programme on Immunization Information Systems,'' WHO/EPI/GEN/89 (Geneva, Switzerland: World Health Organization, 1989).

387. World Health Organization, ''Preventive Tuberculosis Chemotherapy Among Persons Infected With Human Immunodeficiency Virus,'' WHO/TUB/AIDS/90.1 (Genva, Switzerland: World Health Organization, 1990).

388. World Health Organization, ''Tuberculosis Programme and Global Programme on AIDS,'' WHO/TB/92.166 (Geneva, Switzerland: World Health Organization, 1992).

389. Zelinger, G., Medical Advisor, Medicaid Bureau, Health Care Financing Administration, U.S. Department of Health and Human Services, Baltimore, MD, personal communication, Mar. 30, 1993.

390. Zelinger, G., Medical Advisor, Medicaid Bureau, Health Care Financing Administration, U.S. Department of Health and Human Services, Baltimore, MD, personal communication, Apr. 5, 1993.

391. Zelinger, G., Medical Advisor, Medicaid Bureau, Health Care Financing Administration, U.S. Department of Health and Human Services, Baltimore, MD, personal communication, June 25, 1993.

Index

Superintendent of Documents **Publications** Order Form

P3

Order Processing Code:
*7172

☐ **YES**, please send me the following:

Telephone orders (202) 783-3238
To fax your orders (202) 512-2250
Charge your order. It's Easy!

_______ copies of ***The Continuing Challenge of Tuberculosis (160 pages),*** S/N 052-003-01341-0 at $9.50 each.

The total cost of my order is $_________. International customers please add 25%. Prices include regular domestic postage and handling and are subject to change.

(Company or Personal Name) (Please type or print)

(Additional address/attention line)

(Street address)

(City, State, ZIP Code)

(Daytime phone including area code)

(Purchase Order No.)

Please Choose Method of Payment:

☐ Check Payable to the Superintendent of Documents
☐ GPO Deposit Account ☐☐☐☐☐☐☐ — ☐
☐ VISA or MasterCard Account

(Credit card expiration date)

Thank you for your order!

(Authorizing Signature) (9/93)

May we make your name/address available to other mailers? YES ☐ NO ☐

Mail To: New Orders, Superintendent of Documents, P.O. Box 371954, Pittsburgh, PA 15250-7954

THIS FORM MAY BE PHOTOCOPIED

Superintendent of Documents **Publications** Order Form

P3

Order Processing Code:
*7172

☐ **YES**, please send me the following:

Telephone orders (202) 783-3238
To fax your orders (202) 512-2250
Charge your order. It's Easy!

_______ copies of ***The Continuing Challenge of Tuberculosis (160 pages),*** S/N 052-003-01341-0 at $9.50 each.

The total cost of my order is $_________. International customers please add 25%. Prices include regular domestic postage and handling and are subject to change.

(Company or Personal Name) (Please type or print)

(Additional address/attention line)

(Street address)

(City, State, ZIP Code)

(Daytime phone including area code)

(Purchase Order No.)

Please Choose Method of Payment:

☐ Check Payable to the Superintendent of Documents
☐ GPO Deposit Account ☐☐☐☐☐☐☐ — ☐
☐ VISA or MasterCard Account

(Credit card expiration date)

Thank you for your order!

(Authorizing Signature) (9/93)

May we make your name/address available to other mailers? YES ☐ NO ☐

Mail To: New Orders, Superintendent of Documents, P.O. Box 371954, Pittsburgh, PA 15250-7954

THIS FORM MAY BE PHOTOCOPIED